Ralph Schiess

Proteomic Strategy for Cancer Biomarker Discovery

Ralph Schiess

Proteomic Strategy for Cancer Biomarker Discovery

Focus on Cancer Specific Proteins for Diagnostic Purposes

Südwestdeutscher Verlag für Hochschulschriften

Impressum / Imprint

Bibliografische Information der Deutschen Nationalbibliothek: Die Deutsche Nationalbibliothek verzeichnet diese Publikation in der Deutschen Nationalbibliografie; detaillierte bibliografische Daten sind im Internet über http://dnb.d-nb.de abrufbar.

Alle in diesem Buch genannten Marken und Produktnamen unterliegen warenzeichen-, marken- oder patentrechtlichem Schutz bzw. sind Warenzeichen oder eingetragene Warenzeichen der jeweiligen Inhaber. Die Wiedergabe von Marken, Produktnamen, Gebrauchsnamen, Handelsnamen, Warenbezeichnungen u.s.w. in diesem Werk berechtigt auch ohne besondere Kennzeichnung nicht zu der Annahme, dass solche Namen im Sinne der Warenzeichen- und Markenschutzgesetzgebung als frei zu betrachten wären und daher von jedermann benutzt werden dürften.

Bibliographic information published by the Deutsche Nationalbibliothek: The Deutsche Nationalbibliothek lists this publication in the Deutsche Nationalbibliografie; detailed bibliographic data are available in the Internet at http://dnb.d-nb.de.

Any brand names and product names mentioned in this book are subject to trademark, brand or patent protection and are trademarks or registered trademarks of their respective holders. The use of brand names, product names, common names, trade names, product descriptions etc. even without a particular marking in this work is in no way to be construed to mean that such names may be regarded as unrestricted in respect of trademark and brand protection legislation and could thus be used by anyone.

Verlag / Publisher:
Südwestdeutscher Verlag für Hochschulschriften
ist ein Imprint der / is a trademark of
OmniScriptum GmbH & Co. KG
Heinrich-Böcking-Str. 6-8, 66121 Saarbrücken, Deutschland / Germany
Email: info@svh-verlag.de

Herstellung: siehe letzte Seite /
Printed at: see last page
ISBN: 978-3-8381-0639-7

Zugl. / Approved by: Zürich, ETH Zürich, Dissertation, 2008

Copyright © 2009 OmniScriptum GmbH & Co. KG
Alle Rechte vorbehalten. / All rights reserved. Saarbrücken 2009

Abstract

The greatest benefits for patients are likely to be realized from the monitoring and management of early stage disease rather than from treatment of late stage disease. This concept, often called preventive medicine, has been a vision for many years. Among the strategies that have the highest potential to realize the promises of preventive medicine is the detection of prognostic and diagnostic protein signatures in blood plasma and other body fluids. Due to its high sensitivity and high-throughput, mass spectrometry (MS) is the method of choice for the identification and accurate quantification of the proteins contained in complex sample mixtures. Therefore, MS is expected to be a key technology for the discovery of new protein-based biomarkers. Yet despite intensive interest and investment, only a few protein biomarkers are used in clinical practice, and the rate of introduction of new biomarkers into clinical practice is falling. The high complexity and large dynamic range of blood plasma proteins currently prohibits the sensitive and high-throughput profiling of disease and control plasma proteome sample sets large enough to reliably detect disease indicating differences. To circumvent these technological limitations I describe here a new two-stage strategy for the MS assisted discovery, verification and validation of disease biomarkers.

In an initial discovery phase glycoproteins with distinguishable expression patterns in control and diseased tissue are detected and identified. In the second step the proteins identified in the initial phase are subjected to targeted MS analysis in plasma samples, using the highly sensitive and specific selected reaction monitoring (SRM) technology. Since glycosylated proteins, such as those secreted or shed from the cell surface, are likely to reside and persist in blood, the two-stage strategy is focused on the quantification of tissue derived glycoproteins in plasma. The focus on the glyco-proteome not only reduces the complexity of the samples, but also targets an information-rich subproteome which is relevant for remote sensing of diseases in the plasma.

First, I established a strategy for the consecutive analysis of *O*- in addition to *N*-glycoproteins. While the enrichment for *N*-glycoproteins was already established before, I set out to increase the coverage of the glyco-proteome by the selective identification of *O*-glycoproteins. Then, in order to test our hypothesis that the glyco-proteome reflects perturbations in intracellular signaling systems, I investigated the changes in the cell surface glyco-proteome upon stimulation in a well-defined system of *Drosophila melanogaster* cells. Finally, the glycoprotein based biomarker discovery and validation workflow presented here was applied towards the robust and successful identification of human biomarkers for prostate cancer diagnosis. Monitoring the identified set of protein biomarker candidates in the blood plasma of selected patient groups allowed for the sensitive and specific identification of the patient subset with localized prostate cancer. Conclusively, the results presented here outline a new and successful strategy for the remote sensing of protein biomarker candidates in blood by MS-based technologies, which might/should influence decisions on future proteomics based biomarker discovery approaches.

Abbreviations

AQUA	Strategy for the absolute quantification of proteins
BH	Biocytin hydrazide
BPH	Benign prostatic hyperplasia
CA	Cysteamine
CD	Clusters of differentiation
CID	Collision-induced dissociation
CSC	Cell Surface Capturing
cKO	Conditional knock-out
ELISA	Enzyme-Linked ImmunoSorbent Assay
ESI	Electrospray ionization
GO	Gene ontology
HRPC	Hormone refractory prostate cancer
HSPC	Hormone sensitive prostate cancer
ICPL	Isotope coded protein label
IHC	Immunohistochemistry
InR	Insulin receptor (CG18402)
LC	Liquid chromatography
locCaP	Localized prostate cancer
LTQ-FT	Linear ion-trap Fourier transform ion cyclon resonance mass spectrometer
m/z	Mass to charge [Da]
MALDI	Matrix-assisted laser desorption/ionization
MS	Mass spectrometry
MS1 feature	MS1 peak representing a potential peptide ion
MS/MS	Tandem mass spectrometry
N-, O-glycosites	A peptide that is N- or O-glycosylated in the intact protein in its de-glycosylated form
NxS/T motif	Amino acid sequence of asparagine followed by any amino acid (except proline) and either serine or threonine
O-GlcNAc	O-linked β-N-acetylglucosamine
PIN	Prostatic intraepithelial neoplasia
PM	Plasma membrane
PNGase F	N-glycosidase F
PSA	Prostate specific antigen
RT-PCR	Reverse transcribed poly chain reaction
SPEG	Solid-phase extraction of glycopeptides
SRM	Selected reaction monitoring (also called MRM)
TM	Transmembrane
TMA	Tissue microarray
TOF	Time-of-flight
TPP	Trans Proteomic Pipeline

Contents

Abstract	i
Abbreviations	iii
Contents	v
1 Introduction	**1**
1.1 Introduction to proteomics	1
1.1.1 Mass spectrometry based proteomics	2
1.2 Protein biomarkers for preventive and predictive medicine	5
1.2.1 Currently used protein biomarkers and their limitations	6
1.2.2 Protein biomarker discovery strategies and their limitations	7
1.2.3 Performance boundaries for proteomic technologies in biomarker discovery	9
1.3 A role for proteomic technology in all phases of biomarker discovery	10
1.3.1 Generation of biomarker candidate sets by quantitative cell and tissue proteomics	11
1.4 The glyco-proteome enrichment strategy	13
1.4.1 Identification of *N*-glycosites from plasma	14
1.4.2 Selective isolation of *N*-glycosites from cells and tissues	15
1.4.3 Detection of cell/tissue *N*-glycosites in plasma	16
1.4.4 Quantification of *N*-glycosites	17
1.4.5 Selective quantification of tissue derived *N*-glycosites in plasma by targeted mass spectrometry	18
1.5 Motivation of my Ph.D. thesis	19
1.6 References	21
2 Selective isolation and MS-based identification of *O*-linked glycopeptides	**25**
2.1 Authorship	25
2.2 Summary	25
2.3 Introduction	26
2.4 Experimental Procedures	28
2.5 Results	31
2.5.1 Specific glycan release and site mapping of *O*-glycosylation	31
2.5.2 Phosphatase treatment to distinguish *O*-glycosylation and phosphorylation	34
2.5.3 Selective identification of *N*- and *O*-linked glycosites	36
2.5.4 Concurrent identification of *N*- and *O*-glycosites in human serum samples	38
2.6 Discussion	41
2.7 References	42

3 **Phenotyping cells without antibodies: MS identification and quantitation of N-linked cell surface glycoproteins** — 45
  3.1 Authorship — 45
  3.2 Summary — 45
  3.3 Introduction — 46
  3.4 Experimental Procedures — 48
  3.5 Results — 51
    3.5.1 Strategy for the selective identification of cell surface exposed N-glycosites — 51
    3.5.2 The CSC labeling reaction is efficient and selective for glycoproteins — 52
    3.5.3 CSC technology enables the selective MS identification of cell surface glycoproteins — 53
    3.5.4 CSC technology reveals cell surface protein N-glycosite sites and transmembrane protein orientation — 56
    3.5.5 CSC technology is applicable to primary cells, tissues and organs — 57
    3.5.6 CSC technology for quantitative cell surface protein scanning — 58
  3.6 Discussion — 61
  3.7 References — 64

4 **Analysis of cell surface proteome changes via label-free, quantitative mass spectrometry** — 67
  4.1 Authorship — 67
  4.2 Summary — 67
  4.3 Introduction — 68
  4.4 Experimental Procedures — 70
  4.5 Results — 75
    4.5.1 The *D. melanogaster* Kc167 cell surface glyco-proteome atlas — 75
    4.5.2 Reproducible, label-free quantification of the Kc167 cell surface glyco-proteome — 77
    4.5.3 The cell surface proteome changes as a function of cellular state — 79
    4.5.4 Insulin induced internalization of Insulin Receptor (InR) — 82
  4.6 Discussion — 88
  4.7 References — 90

5 **Discovery and validation of protein biomarkers for prostate cancer diagnosis** — 93
  5.1 Authorship — 93
  5.2 Summary — 93
  5.3 Introduction — 94
  5.4 Experimental procedures — 96
  5.5 Results — 101
    5.5.1 Pten-loss induced prostate cancer mouse model — 101
    5.5.2 Proteomic analysis of mouse tissue and serum — 102
    5.5.3 Verification and selection of promising marker candidates — 104
    5.5.4 Verification of marker candidates by targeted MS in mouse serum — 106

5.5.5	ELISA and MS-based validation in human serum	107
5.5.6	Periostin as a potential biomarker for prostate cancer staging	111
5.5.7	Tissue inhibitor of metalloproteinase-1 (TMP-1) as a prognostic marker for survival of patients with hormone refractory prostate cancer (HRPC)	112
5.6	Discussion	113
5.7	References	116

6 Summary of results   **119**

7 Conclusions   **121**

Supplemental Material   **125**

1 Introduction

1.1 Introduction to proteomics

In the past decade numerous genome projects were successfully completed, which had the goal to sequence the whole genome of various organisms. On June 26, 2000, President Clinton and Prime Minister Tony Blair announced in a joint statement the completion of the first survey of the entire human genome – the genetic blueprint for human beings. The completion of the human genome certainly was the highlight of the genomic era[1-3]. This landmark achievement promised to lead to a new era of molecular medicine, an era that would bring new ways to prevent, diagnose, treat and cure disease. Specifically, scientists would now be able to use the human genome to alert patients that they are at risk for certain diseases, reliably predict the course of disease, precisely diagnose disease and ensure the most effective treatment is used and develop new treatments based on molecular mechanisms. However, despite the great success and the progress made in the genetic field, the discovery did not keep its promise and many questions remain open.

One of the big surprises was the relatively low number of about 20'000 human genes detected, only roughly three times more than present in yeast. Even though the human species appears much more complex than yeast, its difference is unlikely to be explained solely by the number of genes. Figure 1.1 (adapted from Lottspeich[4]) gives an enlightening example why genetic data cannot explain many biological processes and functions of an organism.

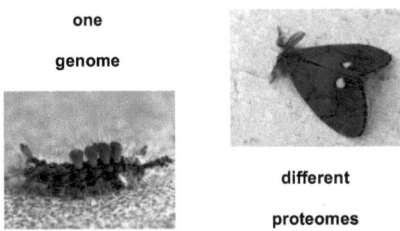

Figure 1.1 Caterpillar and butterfly of *Orgyia antiqua* L. Not only the genome, but in particular the proteins present – the proteome – determine the appearance and state of a biological organism (adapted from Lottspeich[4]).

Despite the fact that each somatic cell of the caterpillar and its counterpart the butterfly possesses the identical genetic information, two totally different phenotypes of the same insect exist. The reason for this is the different translation of the genetic information, i.e. the expression of the individual genes into proteins. The latter are responsible for the biological activity and function of the organism.

Proteomics is the large-scale study of proteins, in particular their structure and function. The proteome is the entirety of proteins expressed in an organism, a cell, an organelle, but also in a tissue or a body fluid, including the modifications made to a particular set of proteins at a given time point under defined conditions. In contrast to the genome, the proteome is much more dynamic, strongly influenced by internal and external factors such as development, differentiation, temperature or stress and thus differs from cell to cell. Furthermore distinct genes are expressed in distinct cell types and many proteins may go through a wide variety of modifications that profoundly affect their activity. For example phosphorylation or glycosylation of certain amino acid residues can influence protein localization, stability, enzymatic activity and protein-protein interactions[5-8].

1.1.1 Mass spectrometry based proteomics

Due to its high sensitivity and high-throughput, mass spectrometry (MS) is the method of choice for the identification and accurate quantification of the proteins contained in complex sample mixtures[9]. Almost 20 years ago, the development of two soft ionization techniques, electrospray ionization (ESI)[10] and matrix-assisted laser desorption/ionization (MALDI)[11], enabled the mass spectrometric analysis of large biomolecules. In 2002, Fenn and Tanaka were awarded with the Nobel Prize for their achievements. Recent advances in MS based proteomics, specifically improved instrumentation, software tools for the analysis of proteomic data sets[12] and emerging, more efficient data collection strategies[13], now routinely lead to the identification of hundreds to thousands of proteins in a single experiment.

MS employs chemical fragmentation of a sample into charged particles (ions) and measures charge and mass of the resulting particles, the ratio of which is deduced by passing the particles through electric and magnetic fields. A mass spectrometer consists of three essential modules: an ion source that transforms the molecules into ionized fragments, a mass analyzer which sorts the ions by their mass to charge ratio (m/z) and a detector that measures the ion intensity and thus provides data for calculating the abundance of each ion fragment present (Figure 1.2). Mass spectrometers mainly differ in respect to the ionization method (ESI or MALDI) and mass analyzers used. The performance and characteristics of a mass spectrometer thus greatly depend on the instrumental setup. The mass accuracy, resolving power, sensitivity and dynamic range of the instrument thereby greatly influence the capability of peptide identification and quantification and detecting modifications thereof at high-throughput[14].

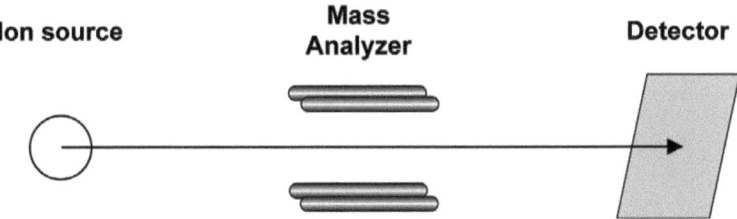

Figure 1.2 A mass spectrometer minimally consists of an ion source where the analytes get ionized. The mass analyzer allows for filtering of the ions according to their mass and finally the detector measures the signal intensity correlating with the analytes abundance.

Tandem mass spectrometry (MS/MS) allows for the sequencing of peptides. The method uses the particular fragmentation pattern generated by peptides. Therefore a certain peptide gets selected in a first mass analyzer. The peptide ions are then stabilized in the collision cell while they collide with an inert gas, causing them to fragment by collision-induced dissociation (CID). The peptide fragments are then sorted in a second mass analyzer and recorded by a detector generating a tandem mass spectrum. This in turn can then be analyzed by bioinformatic means comparing the spectrum to a database of *in silico* generated tandem mass spectra resulting in a peptide identification that in turn can then be used to assign the protein it originated from. Tandem mass spectrometry enables a variety of experimental sequences. One worthwhile to mention is selected reaction monitoring (SRM). Such experiments are used to increase specificity of detection of known peptides. In SRM, the first analyzer allows to filter for a very narrow mass range and the second analyzer monitors for a single user defined peptide fragment ion. Figure 1.3 summarizes the three different MS modes described.

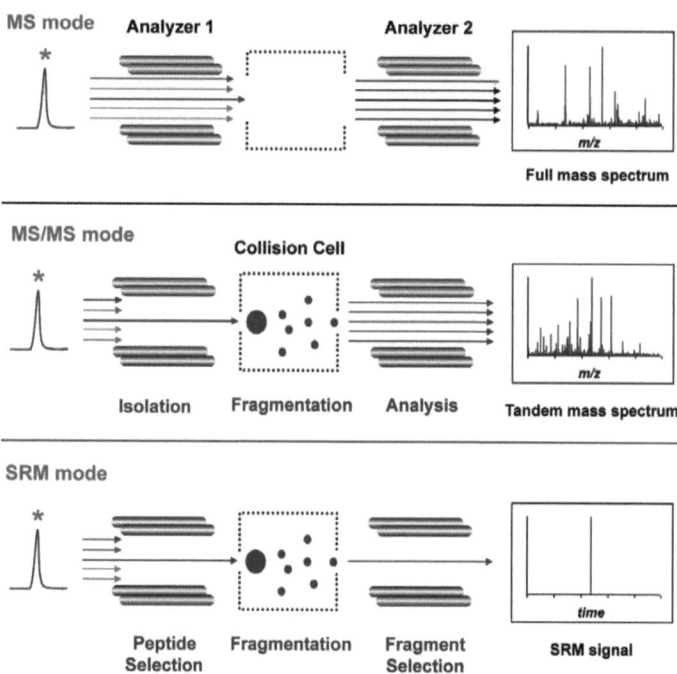

Figure 1.3 Schematic representation of various types of mass spectrometry (MS) experiments. (A) In MS mode only the first mass analyzer is used where the peptide ions are analyzed and a full mass spectrum is generated representing the peptides analyzed at a time. (B) The purpose of MS/MS experiment in proteomics is the generation of fragment ion spectra for the identification of the amino acid sequence of specific peptides. In this experiment, the first analyzer (MS1) is set to a value that selects one specific precursor ion at a time. The selected ion undergoes CID in the collision cell, and the resulting fragments are analyzed by the second analyzer by screening an extended mass range (MS2). This process is repeated for different precursors. (C) SRM consists of a series of short experiments in which one precursor ion and one specific fragment characteristic for that precursor are selected by MS1 and MS2, respectively. Typically, the instrument cycles through a series of transitions (precursor - fragment pair) and records the signal as a function of time (chromatographic elution). SRM is used for the detection of a specific analyte with known fragmentation properties in complex samples.

1.2 Protein biomarkers for preventive and predictive medicine*

The greatest benefits for patients are likely to be realized from the monitoring and management of early stage disease rather than from treatment of late stage disease. This concept, often called preventive medicine, has been a vision for many years. Recent technological advancements along with the information generated by the human genome project offer great hope for making the early detection of diseases a reality within the next few years in many disease settings[15-17].

Among the strategies that have the highest potential to realize the promises of preventive medicine is the detection of prognostic and diagnostic protein signatures in blood plasma** and other body fluids. It has been shown that personalized molecular gene expression signatures can be detected in tissues and that these signatures can aid clinicians to diagnose early stage disease, stratify similar pathologies, and to distinguish those diseases which respond to current therapy from those that do not[18-21]. As an example, in 2007, the FDA cleared the first multivariate molecular test that profiles genetic activity. It is a breast cancer specific molecular prognostic test which correlates the expression pattern of 21 genes in paraffin-embedded tumor tissue probes with the likelihood of distant reoccurrence in patients with node-negative, tamoxifen-treated breast cancer[22]. Although the test is of highly predictive value it requires the complicated and costly clinical extraction of selective breast tissue samples.

Unfortunately, most human tissues are difficult to access and it is unlikely that human tissue will be routinely analyzed in large populations for the presence of such predictive gene expression signatures. In contrast, human blood is easily accessible for sampling and contains informational cues from all organs which it is contacting through a network of arteries, veins and capillaries. During its journey through the cardiovascular system blood has been shown to collect molecular cues consisting of proteins secreted, shed or otherwise released from tissues[23, 24]. Therefore, the quantitative protein composition of blood plasma contains information about the state of organs and the whole organism in health and disease - an informational network which needs to be deciphered to allow for remote sensing of specific diseases. The mapping of this informational network requires robust, reproducible and sensitive measurements of single protein markers or selected protein panels. Such protein panels can be thought to reflect the perturbed molecular networks in the disease microenvironment. The task for a successful blood biomarker strategy therefore involves the analysis of the disease perturbed cellular networks, the identification of cellular proteins that indicate the state of the perturbed networks and their detection and quantification in blood plasma.

---

* The following part of the introduction is extracted from a recent review from Schiess, R. et al., *Molecular Oncology* **3**, 33-44 (2009).

** The term plasma is used to indicate serum or plasma

1.2 Protein biomarkers for preventive and predictive medicine

1.2.1 Currently used protein biomarkers and their limitations

Initial attempts to use the information contained in the blood proteome for early diagnosis were focused on the detection and quantitative measurement of single protein markers via affinity reagents. This is exemplified by the best known plasma biomarker, prostate specific antigen (PSA). Despite its now well recognized limited specificity for the detection of prostate cancer, PSA continues to be the most widely used tumor marker in the world. The discovery of PSA is beset with controversy as different researchers discovered it independently using immunological techniques, resulting in different names for the same marker[25]. Originally, PSA was of interest for immunological reasons. Tissue specific antigens were believed to be targets for specific antibodies in order to destroy cancer[26]. Later PSA was also suggested as forensic evidence in cases of rape[27]. Only in 1987, some 27 years after the first publication, Stamey et al.[28] suggested in a landmark study to use PSA as a marker for prostate cancer.

PSA was found to be specifically expressed in prostate tissue and to be secreted into the blood stream at elevated levels upon disease progression. A second reason for using PSA as a tumor marker was the availability of specific antibodies for standardized and affordable ELISA blood tests. A second well-known example of a single protein biomarker is the Her2/neu proto-oncogene (CD340). This membrane bound receptor tyrosine kinase exemplifies the way scientists in the 1980s attempted to uncover new cancer-causing oncogenes. By over expressing genes of interest, the effect of potential oncogenes on cancer induction or development was assayed. In one such study the Her2/neu gene was found to cause breast cancer in rats[29]. Later, it was found to be amplified in up to 30% of invasive breast cancers and its over-expression to be associated with a poor prognosis[30]. Elevated plasma levels of CD340 are therefore used as an indicator for higher aggressiveness in breast cancer[31]. Her2/neu is not only used as a biomarker, but also as a target of trastuzumab (Herceptin) in anti-cancer therapy[32]. Both examples showcase single proteins which can "leak" from diseased tissue into the bloodstream and are indicative for a disease if detected at elevated plasma levels. Unfortunately, neither PSA nor Her2/neu, nor for that matter any other single protein biomarker in clinical use, have sufficiently high sensitivity and specificity to predict the development of a particular form of disease and to accurately detect it at an early stage. In the Prostate Cancer Prevention Trial (PCPT), among 5'112 men, PSA level > 4 ng/ml had specificity of 93% and a rather low sensitivity of 24%[33], while a study by Cook et al.[34] revealed that at an upper limit at 15 ng/ml of Her2/neu the specificity for normal breast was 98% and the sensitivity for breast cancer stage IV disease was only 40%.

Therefore, additional test parameters are needed in combination with current biomarker tests to increase their performance. A panel of disease-specific protein biomarkers is thought to be necessary to narrow down diagnosis and treatment options, and reliable strategies for the discovery of such panels

1 - Introduction

need to be developed. Furthermore, both examples cited above highlight another major limitation for current protein biomarker measurements. Without suitable antibodies or other affinity reagents to sensitively and unambiguously detect and quantify the respective proteins, their validation and use as protein biomarkers has been substantially limited.

1.2.2 Protein biomarker discovery strategies and their limitations

Most clinically relevant biomarkers have been discovered serendipitously, as already mentioned in the case of PSA and Her2/neu, or via a circuitous route of trial and error. Substances thought to be associated with a certain disease were further investigated in several directions[35]. For example, in 1847 Bence Jones detected large quantities of a particular protein in the urine of a multiple myeloma patient[36]. More than a hundred years later the protein was identified as a free antibody light chain produced by the tumor[37] that was also present in blood plasma[38]. It was a 152 years after its first discovery that in the year 1998 the FDA approved a routine immunodiagnostic test for the protein as a diagnostic marker for multiple myeloma. Clearly, such non-directed biomarker discovery efforts, while occasionally successful, lack the efficiency to be of general utility for medicine.

The emerging field of proteomics with its objective to comprehensively identify and quantify proteomes immediately raised high expectations for plasma biomarker discovery[39]. Most biomarker discovery studies based on proteomics to date attempted to detect proteins specifically associated with disease by the comparative profiling of plasma proteomes (or specific fractions thereof) of healthy control and disease affected donors. Several proteomic techniques have been applied for this purpose, including two-dimensional gel electrophoresis[40], SELDI-TOF MS[41], label-free LC-MS pattern comparison[42], LC-MS/MS shotgun analysis[43, 44], and protein array methods[45]. However, these purely discovery-driven studies have achieved only modest success. While these methods, either by themselves or in combination, have achieved substantial progress in the quantity and quality of data generated, every presently known plasma proteomic method today still only samples a relatively small fraction of the proteome that mostly consists of the relatively highly expressed proteins. Both the large dynamic concentration range of up to 12 orders of magnitude for plasma proteins but also the presence of very high abundance proteins such as serum albumin (35-50 mg/ml) and immunoglobulins (5-18 mg/ml) which mask the lower abundance plasma proteins present major challenges for comprehensive plasma proteome analysis, especially for proteins below the microgram per milliliter concentration limit[46]. The discrepancy between the sensitivity of present proteomics methods and the requirements for biomarker discovery is illustrated in Figure 1.4. The figure indicates the concentration of proteins identified by the HUPO plasma proteome collaborative study[47] and that of currently used plasma biomarkers[48]. It is apparent that the concentration ranges of the two populations barely overlap, suggesting that it is unlikely that the continued application of the same methods in further studies will discover new biomarkers. The presently used proteomics methods mainly sample so called classical plasma proteins in the range of µg/ml to mg/ml. In contrast, the PSA concentration in blood plasma of healthy individuals is around 2 ng/ml[49, 50], and the blood plasma concentration of Her2/neu is in the range of 10 ng/ml, about one order of magnitude higher than for PSA[51]. Both plasma biomarkers are thus situated in the lower region of currently known plasma protein abundance levels and the same applies to other plasma biomarkers known today. Thus, future biomarker discovery technologies have to be able to reliably detect plasma proteins in the low ng/ml concentration range, or even below the ng/ml range.

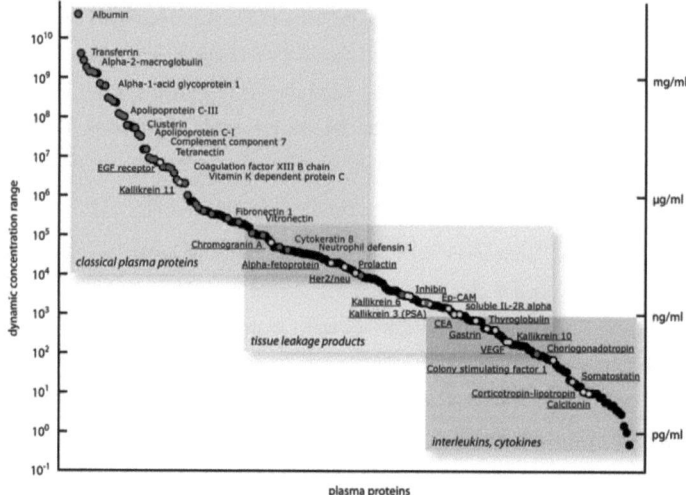

Figure 1.4 Depicted are the plasma protein concentration as described by Anderson et al.[46]. The proteins can be grouped in three main categories (classical plasma proteins, tissue leakage products, interleukins/cytokines). Red dots indicate proteins that were identified by the HUPO plasma proteome initiative[47] and yellow dots represent currently utilized biomarkers[48].

Because currently used LC-MS-based proteomic methods have great difficulty to analyze low abundance proteins, numerous protein and/or peptide separation methods have been used to reduce plasma sample complexity and thus to increase sensitivity of detection in the thus generated fractions. The most common protein fractionation methods use size fractionation by gel electrophoresis or chromatography. While protein fractionation methods performed upstream of a mass spectrometric shotgun analysis have to be performed offline, peptide separation based on hydrophobicity can be

1 - Introduction

achieved online and is therefore easier to automate. Although sample fractionation is the key to a higher number and quality for protein identifications, in the context of a biomarker discovery effort such techniques can be problematic for mainly two reasons. First, sample fractionation increases the number of samples to be analyzed, which is time and labor intensive to a degree that routine measurements of larger patient groups become prohibitive. Second, variations along a multi-step protein separation workflow, e.g. the slightly different distribution of specific proteins in collected fractions, will add another level of bioinformatic complexity towards the detection of disease related patterns. Another popular strategy to achieve higher sensitivity in MS assisted plasma proteome analyses has been the selective removal of high-abundance proteins such as albumin and the various forms of immunoglobulins by selective immunodepletion. A study published by Echan et al.[52] showed that effective depletion of six abundant proteins resulted in the ability to load larger equivalent amounts of plasma into downstream separation workflows including 2-D gels, leading to a more in depth plasma proteome characterization. The removal of the six most abundant plasma proteins depletes 85% of the total plasma protein resulting in an estimated five-fold enrichment of a potential biomarker[53]. Another immunodepletion LC column removes 99% of the 20 most high abundance plasma proteins representing 97% of the proteome giving rise to an up to 20-fold enrichment as stated by the manufacturer (Sigma-Aldrich). Despite these improvements, the currently used MS assisted biomarker discovery efforts still lack the needed sensitivity and the throughput required to identify biomarker candidates in the low ng/ml concentration range by the comparative analysis of multiple samples.

Based on these observations it can be concluded that the next generation proteomics-based protein biomarker discovery strategies need improved analytical sensitivity, robustness and sample throughput in order to reliably detect tissue specific protein patterns in plasma with high specificity. Moreover, special attention has to be paid to the time consuming and labor intensive validation of the large datasets produced by these methods in a relatively short time, an issue that so far has been neglected in most studies as pointed out in recent reviews[54, 55].

1.2.3 Performance boundaries for proteomic technologies in biomarker discovery

In the segment above the limitations of current proteomic methods for protein biomarker discovery were discussed. Here the performance boundaries that have likely to be matched for a method to be successful are examined.

The accessible human body fluids such as plasma, urine, ascites, semen, saliva, seminal plasma and cerebrospinal fluid are thought to contain tens of thousands of different proteins spanning more than 10 orders of magnitude in abundance. To comprehensively analyze such samples at the required sample throughput a proteomic technology has to meet a number of so far unmet requirements. First, the technology has to have the sensitivity to identify and quantify minute amounts of proteins in plasma to a concentration of at least low ng/ml, i.e. seven orders of magnitude in concentration below albumin. In that regard good signal to noise ratios are critical to exclude artifactual results. This is particularly challenging if the concentration range assayed exceeds the dynamic range of the MS platform used[56]. Second, any proteomic platform for the discovery of candidate disease protein biomarkers must have the capacity for the automated, repetitive and reproducible analysis of hundreds of patient samples in a relatively short time period to achieve sufficient statistical power to be clinically useful. Third, clinically relevant diagnostic markers require both high sensitivity and specificity. To achieve this goal, any proteomic platform in a biomarker discovery workflow requires robustness in the sense that repetitive measurements achieve coefficients of variance in the low single digit range, and fourth, the assay that measures the protein or sets of proteins in question needs to be portable between laboratories in a way that guarantees comparable results obtained in different studies.

Apart from the technological challenges, the quest for standardized protein biomarkers as measurable disease predicting indicators is further complicated by the genetic variation among individuals[57]. This genetic variation causes measurable protein abundance changes within the plasma of individuals that are independent of any disease state, making it difficult to define "normal" protein levels. Furthermore, one has to consider that the plasma proteome is dynamic over time and a function of a multitude of factors (daytime, age, sex, etc.). Therefore, disease related protein abundance changes especially in the onset of a disease can be buried within normal plasma protein fluctuations within the individuals tested[58]. On top of this, even at the single protein level an array of protein modifications such as posttranslational modifications as well as point mutations frequently occur expanding the potential variation among patients boundlessly[59]. In order to circumvent some of the above mentioned challenges at least in the biomarker discovery phase genetically stable mouse models of disease could simplify the initial protein biomarker candidate selection[60].

1.3 A role for proteomic technology in all phases of biomarker discovery

The process of identifying new protein biomarkers can be mainly divided into four major phases as suggested by Rifai et al.[56]. In the initial discovery phase, proteins of differential abundance in plasma are identified and classified. Subsequently, promising candidates are qualified in a second phase and a subset of these verified in a third phase. In the last phase, the surviving candidates are validated as potential biomarkers by using a specifically developed high-throughput assay, usually ELISA. During this four-step biomarker discovery process, the number of samples that need to be analyzed increases while the number of potential biomarker candidates decreases from initially hundreds to a few candidates. These

1 - Introduction

remaining candidates must be verified and validated by showing discriminative power in clinical studies among large cohorts of cancer positive and negative patients. The rationale for choosing this path of progressive attrition of biomarker candidates is rooted in the practical challenge to quantify large numbers of proteins in large numbers of samples, rather than in fundamental considerations. In fact, in an ideal scenario all the putative biomarkers would be subjected to rigorous validation in large sample sets, thus avoiding the application of arbitrary rules to reduce the candidate pool at each step.

Until very recently mass spectrometry has been used almost exclusively for the identification of potential biomarker candidates, whereas their verification and validation has traditionally been carried out by higher throughput affinity methods. Emerging new MS-based analytical platforms with increased selectivity and sensitivity have now the capacity to be instrumental not only in the initial phase of biomarker discovery but also for the follow-up studies in clinical settings. Multiplexed measurements of biomarker candidates via targeted MS methods such as selected reaction monitoring (SRM; also referred to as multiple reaction monitoring, MRM) have the potential to speed-up the expensive and time-consuming biomarker verification and validation phases. Therefore, the application of emerging targeted mass spectrometry-based proteomics methods with their proven ability to reliably and sensitively detect and quantify pre-determined sets of proteins in complex samples will be instrumental for protein biomarker discovery as well as qualification, verification and validation, respectively.

1.3.1 Generation of biomarker candidate sets by quantitative cell and tissue proteomics

Above the challenges in identifying protein biomarker candidates by comparative plasma proteomics were discussed. Compared to detecting meaningful disease related protein differences in plasma the challenges of identifying proteins that differentiate cancerous and normal cells and tissues are significantly reduced. This is due to the fact that the protein concentration range in tissue is expected to be lower than in blood which facilitates the measurement of a higher percentage of the proteome in a single analysis[61, 62]. Cell lines have the additional advantage that in most cases the amount of sample needed for MS analysis is not limited which makes cell lysates compatible with extensive fractionation schema, further increasing the likelihood of discovering proteins of lower abundance. A key benefit of tissue samples is the fact that the differential proteome profiles can be directly investigated at the origin of the disease. Therefore, disease indicating protein concentration differences are expected to be more pronounced in suitable tissue samples compared to the blood stream where the relevant tissue derived proteins are expected to be detected after significant dilution. Assuming that a protein gets secreted from the prostate into the blood, the protein would be a thousand times more concentrated in the tissue by simply comparing the volume of prostate and plasma.

1.3 A role for proteomic technology in all phases of biomarker discovery

In turn, protein abundance ratio changes in the tissue compared to blood are also expected to be higher and thus easier to detect with the MS-based quantification strategies currently available.

For the detection of biomarker candidates from tissue, it is critical to start out with a well-defined group of samples, i.e. the disease samples must be classified clearly and differentiated from the control group. For statistical analysis, at least three independent samples of each condition need to be available to account for biological variations. In order to follow the progression of the disease, it is also beneficial to have defined samples at different stages of disease development, as pointed out earlier. Conditional gene knock-in/out models leading to a specific disease phenotype are excellent systems as starting points for biomarker discovery efforts, provided that they closely recapitulate the known human disease stages. Such systems offer the opportunity for sampling at the very early stage of the disease where the genetic preposition for the disease is present but no disease-specific phenotype is detectable. Upon the possible sampling at the onset of the disease, genetic model systems also allow for consistent sampling at different disease stages.

Cancerous diseases are categorized according to the following stages as defined by the National Cancer Institute (NCI)[63]: Stage 0 – the amount of cancerous cells is relatively small and constrained to the organ within which it developed. Stage I-III –From stage I to III, the cancer gets more extensive and the tumor size increases. Sometimes nearby lymph nodes contain cancer cells and the cancer spreads to organs adjacent to the primary tumor. Stage IV – the cancer has spread from where it started to another body organ, such as the liver, bones or lungs (See Table 1.1). Thus, a valid animal model should recapitulate the different stages so that valuable conclusions can be drawn from the discovery phase. Nowadays, cancer progression is described using TNM staging and various disease specific grading such as the Gleason score for prostate cancer[64]. In the TNM staging system the disease is assessed using a combination of tumor size or depth (T), lymph node spread (N), and presence or absence of metastases (M)[65].

Table 1.1 Description of the different stages used TNM classification as defined by NCI[63].

Stage	Definition
Stage 0	Carcinoma in situ (early cancer that is present only in the layer of cells in which it began).
Stage I, Stage II, and Stage III	Higher numbers indicate more extensive disease: greater tumor size, and/or spread of the cancer to nearby lymph nodes and/or organs adjacent to the primary tumor.
Stage IV	The cancer has spread to another organ.

1 - Introduction 13

Valid disease and benign control tissue samples, or cell lines representing different disease states are crucial resources for MS-assisted biomarker discovery, especially if used with new mass spectrometry-based workflows of increased throughput and sensitivity.

In the following, a new biomarker discovery strategy based upon the directed analysis of glycoproteins in plasma is described. The approach presented circumvents most of the above mentioned limitations and supports the multiplexed measurement of protein targets with increased sensitivity and high quantitative accuracy, and the throughput required for discovering and evaluating new biomarker candidates.

1.4 The glyco-proteome enrichment strategy

In searching for a method having the potential to detect tissue-specific protein signatures in blood plasma, methods for the selective analysis of de-glycosylated peptides that are N-glycosylated in the intact protein, termed solid-phase extraction of N-glycopeptides (SPEG)[66] have been developed. These peptides are referred to as N-glycosites. The focus on the sub proteome of N-glycosites is based on the fact that most proteins that are localized on the cell surface or secreted from cells are glycosylated[67]. Our working assumption was that disease-associated glycoproteins secreted or shed from cell surfaces, or otherwise released from tissue, might be detectable by remote detection in the blood stream. The potential of such a strategy focusing onto the N-glycosite subproteome was further supported by a re-evaluation of a list of current plasma biomarkers published by Polanski et al.[48]. Thirty out of the 38 proteins within the list of protein biomarkers currently used in the clinic and thus a vast majority is known to be glycosylated (Table 1.2).

Table 1.2 List of markers in clinical use including their plasma concentration in controls and status of glycosylation.

Protein Names	Plasma concentration in controls pg/ml	Clinical Markers	SwissProt # (human)	Glycosylation
Alkaline phosphatase, placental type		√	P05187	yes
Alpha-fetoprotein	2.00E+04	√	P02771	yes
CA 125		√	Q8WXI7	yes
CA 15.3		√	P15941	yes
CA 19.9		√	x	yes
CA 27.29		√	x	yes
CA 72-4		√	x	yes
Carcinoembryonic antigen	1.00E+03	√	P06731	yes
Choriogonadotropin beta chain	1.00E+02	√	P01233	yes

(continued)

1.4 The glyco-proteome enrichment strategy

Table 1.2 (continued)

Protein Names	Plasma concentration in controls pg/ml	Clinical Markers	SwissProt # (human)	Glycosylation
Chromogranin A (parathyroid secretory protein 1)	6.50E+04	√	P10645	yes
Colony stimulating factor 1 (macrophage)	7.00E+01	√	P09603	yes
Complement factor H related protein		√	Q03591	yes
Corticotropin-lipotropin contains ACTH	1.10E+01	√	P01189	yes
Epidermal growth factor receptor	6.94E+06	√	P00533	yes
Follicle-stimulating hormone		√	P01225	yes
Hepatocyte growth factor	2.00E+02	√	P14210	yes
Inhibin	3.00E+03	√	P05111	yes
Kallikrein 10	4.39E+02	√	O43240	yes
Kallikrein 11	2.15E+06	√	Q9UBX7	yes
Kallikrein 3 (prostate specific antigen)	1.86E+03	√	P07288	yes
Kallikrein 5		√	Q9Y337	yes
Kallikrein 6	2.90E+03	√	Q92876	yes
Kallikrein 7		√	P49862	yes
Kallikrein 8		√	O60259	yes
Luteinizing hormone-releasing hormone receptor		√	P22888	yes
Mesothelin		√	Q13421	yes
MK-1 protein, Ep-CAM	2.00E+03	√	P16422	yes
OVX1		√	x	yes
Prolactin	1.60E+04	√	P01236	yes
Soluble IL-2R alpha	1.42E+03	√	P01589	yes
Somatotropin growth factor, growth hormone	4.00E+02	√	P01241	yes
Thyroglobulin	1.00E+03	√	P01266	yes
V-erb-b2, Her2/neu	1.12E+04	√	P04626	yes
Vascular endothelial growth factor A, VEGF	2.01E+02	√	P15692	yes
Calcitonin	1.00E+01	√	P01258	no
Estrogen receptor 1		√	P03372	no
Gastrin	6.90E+02	√	P01350	no
Insulin		√	P01308	no
Parathyroid hormone-related protein		√	P12272	no
Progesterone receptor		√	P06401	no
Somatostatin	2.00E+01	√	P61278	no
Vasoactive intestinal peptide		√	P01282	no

1.4.1 Identification of N-glycosites from plasma

Protein glycosylation has long been recognized as a common co-translational modification. Typically, carbohydrates are linked to serine or threonine residues (O-linked glycosylation) or to asparagine residues (N-linked glycosylation). N-linked glycosylation sites generally fall into the NxS/T sequence motif in which x denotes any amino acid except proline. In contrast, a consensus primary amino acid sequence for

1 - Introduction

O-glycosylation sites has not been identified. Glycoproteins can be enriched either via lectins[68] leaving the carbohydrate structure intact or via coupling to a hydrazide support[69]. In this case, the carbohydrates are oxidized with sodium periodate and the aldehydes formed for affinity purification can be covalently coupled to a hydrazide containing support as described by Bayer/Wilcheck[69] and Zhang et al.[66]. For subsequent mass-spectrometric identification, *N*-glycosites can be specifically released from the solid support by PNGase F. The catalytic action of the enzyme also converts the formerly glycosylated asparagine residue via deamidation into aspartic acid. This enzymatic conversion leads to a mass shift of 0.98 Da which can readily be detected by high mass accuracy mass spectrometers. The MS detectable mass shift improves the confidence of the peptide identification and unambiguously identifies the asparagine residue(s) to which the carbohydrate was linked in the intact protein.

1.4.2 Selective isolation of *N*-glycosites from cells and tissues

While soluble glycoproteins in plasma can be readily isolated and analyzed, glycoproteins embedded in cellular membranes within tissues are more difficult to isolate and identify. Typically, the tissue/cell samples have to be homogenized prior to glycoprotein isolation, or a cell free supernatant of collagenase digested tissues has to be used for *N*-glycosites extraction as described by Tian et al.[70].

To isolate the *N*-glycosites specifically from cell surface glycoproteins a variant of the SPEG method has been developed, the cell surface capturing (CSC) method, where glycoproteins can be selectively enriched from the plasma membrane of intact, living cells[71]. CSC allows for the selective isolation, identification and quantification of cell surface glycoproteins, and the MS data reveals a snapshot of the cell surface protein landscape at the time of labeling. The selective and multiplexed identification of cell surface glycoproteins of a specific cell type is especially interesting for targeted therapeutic approaches. Almost two-thirds of the currently used therapeutic targets are among these plasma membrane proteins[72].

In contrast to the identification of *N*-glycosites, *O*-glycosites are more difficult to study mainly due to a lack of a consensus sequence around the carbohydrate attachment site and the lack of an enzyme analogous to PNGase F that generally removes *O*-linked carbohydrate from the glycoprotein. Thus, chemical approaches for the efficient deglycosylation of *O*-glycosites in complex samples, such as β-elimination are currently being explored albeit with limited success so far.

To date a suite of methods for the specific MS identification of *N*-glycosites from the cell surface, complete cells, tissue and plasma has been developed. All these methods have been extensively applied towards the identification of *N*-glycosites from human and murine cells, tissue and plasma. In particular, plasma samples were extensively fractionated in several dimensions on the protein and peptide level to reach an extensive coverage of the human plasma glyco-proteome[73]. The identified peptides/proteins were consistently annotated and imported into the established database UniPep (http://www.unipep.org), a publicly accessible repository for N-glycosites[74]. UniPep protein entries are annotated by the number of times a particular N-glycosite was observed including relevant meta information about the source of origin and associated parameters which are critical for biomarker discovery efforts. UniPep is part of the PeptideAtlas project (http://www.peptideatlas.org) which comprises a growing publicly accessible database of peptides not restricted to N-glycosites that were detected in many MS-based proteomic studies[75] and an instance of the PeptideAtlas database[76]. Such databases are cornerstones for the future target selection of peptides in emerging MS-assisted biomarker studies relying on directed proteomic workflows as reviewed by E. Deutsch et al.[77].

1.4.3 Detection of cell/tissue N-glycosites in plasma

As pointed out earlier, it was assumed initially that proteins released by tissue (secreted, shed or otherwise released) into the blood stream could be detected in plasma for remote sensing of the state of specific cells/tissues in health and disease. Our approach, the comprehensive analysis of N-glycosites seemed to be ideally suited for the remote sensing of such signatures, due to the fact that glycoproteins and therefore N-glycosites are an information rich subproteome with the benefit of a reduced proteome complexity. In initial studies Zhang et al. therefore set out to determine whether N-glycosites identified in various cell and tissue samples were represented in the plasma by comparing the MS identified N-glycosites within the relational database UniPep, being the perfect tool for such a comparison. As shown in Figure 1.5a, a large number of N-glycosites and proteins that were identified from lymphocytes, bladder, prostate, breast and liver were also detected in the respective plasma samples[24]. The data provided proof that it is possible to identify cellular N-glycosites in the plasma. However, the data represent only an indirect proof of our concept, since the N-glycosites identified within the plasma cannot be attributed at this point directly to the cell or tissue of origin. For example, 202 unique N-glycosites in both prostate tissue and plasma were identified. Of these, 96 likely to originate from classic plasma proteins, 94 are likely to have originated from prostate tissue and cells, and the remaining 12 originated from hypothetical proteins with no protein information to determine their source.

Nevertheless, a subsequent comparison of N-glycosites identified from SK-BR-3 breast cancer cells and Jurkat T lymphocytes by using the CSC technology with prostate N-glycosites and plasma identified N-glycosites provided further evidence for our concept. As shown in Figure 1.5a, 77 peptides identified from lymphocytes and 286 peptides from breast cancer cells were also detected in plasma. When peptides identified from lymphocytes and breast cancer cells with the peptides identified from prostate tissue were compared, only 5 peptides were found to be common to all three samples (Figure 1.5b). This indicates that N-glycosites derived from cells and tissues can be detected in plasma and might be linked to their specific cell/tissue of origin. Collectively these data indicate that cell/tissue-derived N-glycosites can be specifically detected in plasma via newly developed N-glycosite capturing workflows in combination with MS/MS.

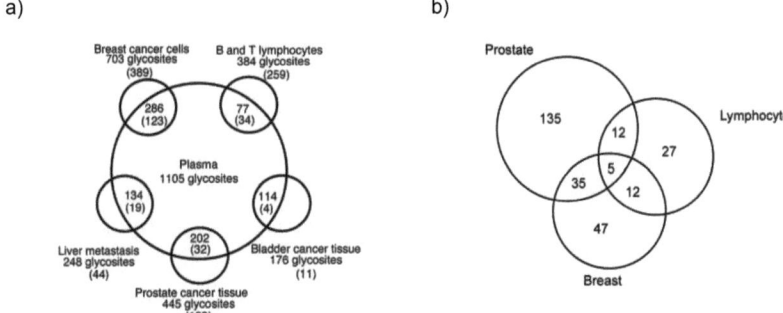

Figure 1.5 Schematic diagram of analysis of N-linked N-glycosites from tissues/cells and plasma. Cell surface proteins and secreted proteins from tissues/cells and plasma are processed using glycopeptide capture method, glycopeptides are analyzed by mass spectrometry and identified by SEQUEST search. The identified peptides and proteins from tissues/cells and plasma are compared and the tissue/cell specific proteins are identified. Figure was adapted from Zhang et al.[24].

1.4.4 Quantification of N-glycosites

Peptides extracted from either cells, tissue or plasma can be MS quantified by using a number of stable isotope labeling technologies as reviewed by Bantscheff et al. and Mueller et al.[78, 79]. The introduction of stable isotopes through stable isotope labeling into protein samples has the advantage that after the labeling process the samples can be processed in parallel and thus the variability among the samples can be limited[80]. However, isotopic labeling increases sample complexity due the differential labeling and combining the samples. Furthermore, the number of samples that can be compared directly is limited by the number of isotopic labels (ICAT/2; iTRAQ/4-8; SILAC/3). In contrast, recently emerging label-free quantification workflows using either spectral counting[81, 82] or peptide elution ion trace profiles[83, 84] have the advantage that they are not limited in the number of samples analyzed, rather by the sample amount itself. Although label-free quantification of peptides reduces the individual sample manipulation steps, which is beneficial for pattern detection, the workflow requires the independent MS analysis of the samples. This in turn requires sophisticated computational tools for the alignment of the MS runs and the subsequent quantification of peptide ratios. Because this approach seemed suitable for the bioinformatic

MS analysis of clinical samples in a high-throughput manner we developed the software SuperHirn[84] and applied label-free quantitative proteomics to the detection of N-glycosites. The experiments revealed that the combination of label-free quantification and SuperHirn is a robust quantitative technology platform to profile N-glycosites[85].

1.4.5 Selective quantification of tissue derived N-glycosites in plasma by targeted mass spectrometry

To identify N-glycosites with diagnostic information in plasma it is necessary to screen multiple plasma samples for the presence of the respective proteins in a selective, parallel and absolute quantitative fashion. This can be accomplished by combining the previously generated knowledge about N-glycosites with targeted MS assisted via SRM. The requirements for targeted MS are twofold. First, one needs to know which proteins/peptides are to be targeted and secondly, a selective SRM assay has to be established for the absolute quantification of the protein of interest. The necessary information about individual N-glycosites required for establishing the SRM assay can be retrieved either by searching the UniPep (or PeptideAtlas) databases, or bioinformatically estimated using a suite of software tools[86-88]. For each protein to be measured at least one peptide which is unique for the selected protein, a so called proteotypic peptide, has to be chosen[87]. By measuring only selected proteotypic peptides, the presence or absence of a protein and its abundance, respectively, can be definitively established. Sets of proteotypic peptides can be detected and quantified very precisely by using triple quadrupole MS or triple quadrupole/linear ion trap hybrid MS instruments by applying SRM. Highly sensitive and selective SRM analyses are performed by monitoring fragmentation channels specific to each peptide of interest[89]. From a technical point of view, a precursor ion is selected by the first quadrupole, fragmented in the second quadrupole and characteristic fragment ions of the precursor are detected and counted upon selection in the third quadrupole by a sensitive detector. The SRM technology ensures higher selectivity by eliminating co-eluting interferences and thus allows for the detection of low abundance components. This gained increase in sensitivity compared to shotgun MS workflows is critical for the success of MS assisted biomarker discovery efforts. Absolute quantification of the selected peptides can be performed by concomitantly monitoring the fragmentations of the corresponding isotopically labeled peptides that are added to the plasma samples prior to their analysis. A linear response over a wide concentration range of at least five orders of magnitude was observed by Stahl-Zeng et al.[90]. The detection limit for peptides present in the mixture was around 30 atmol (i.e. amount actually injected into the LC/MS system), which translates to a protein concentration in the original plasma sample of some 100 pg/ml. However, it is important to note that this sensitivity could only be achieved by reducing the sample complexity through N-glycosite capturing. Similar results cannot be achieved to date by measuring whole plasma samples due

1 - Introduction

to sample complexity in combination with signal to noise issues in available MS instrumentation. Apart from the increased sensitivity of N-glycosite SRM assays compared to shotgun proteomic workflows, such a strategy enables the quantitative measurement of currently up to 500 peptides per MS run in a selective, repetitive and automated manner[91].

1.5 Motivation of my Ph.D. thesis

The greatest benefits to the well-being of mankind will come, not from the treatment of highly advanced disease, but from the monitoring and management of early stage disease. Proteomics has raised great expectation in the discovery of new biomarkers. Yet despite intensified interest and investment, few novel biomarkers are used in clinical practice, and their rate of introduction is falling. Indeed, since 1998, the rate of introduction of new protein analytes approved by the US Food and Drug Administration has fallen to an average of one per year. The reasons for this disjunction are manifold and reflect the long and difficult path from candidate discovery to clinical assay, and the lack of coherent and comprehensive processes (pipelines) for biomarker development[56].

Currently used MS assisted biomarker discovery platforms are not sensitive enough and lack throughput. Sensitivity is mainly hampered by the huge complexity of the protein samples obtained from human body fluids. Thus the goal of my Ph.D. thesis was to show that MS could play a role in all phases of biomarker discovery. To circumvent current limitations, I will enrich for a subproteome, the glyco-proteome. The selective enrichment of glycoproteins allows for the detection of low abundant proteins in complex protein samples such as blood since the high abundant non-glycoprotein serum albumin is neglected and only a few peptides, the N- or O-glycosites, per protein are isolated and analyzed by LC-MS/MS. Furthermore, the selective focus on this particular subproteome allows for the discovery driven identification of glycoproteins in tissue and cell culture followed by the targeted analysis of these secreted or otherwise released proteins in blood plasma. Therefore SRM assays have to be established for N-glycosites originating from those tissue-derived glycoproteins.

Importantly, new biomarkers must outperform currently available markers. To do so, I will show that proteins can be reliably and routinely detected at the low ng/ml range. Current MS techniques can still be improved in terms of sample throughput and reproducibility as well as software tools for automated SRM scheduling need to be developed and improved. Furthermore, resources for the community such as an SRM atlas need to be built up.

I strongly believe that the strategy to be applied here by choosing targeted MS would speed up biomarker discovery (Figure 1.6). Furthermore I will demonstrate that targeted MS in combination with

1.5 Motivation of my Ph.D. thesis

solid phase enrichment of N-glycosites reaches required sensitivity and throughput due to the fact that up to 500 candidates can be monitored in parallel. Therefore this approach finally has significant advantages in the speed of assay development compared to current ELISA techniques and thus will play an important role in further preclinical biomarker evaluation studies.

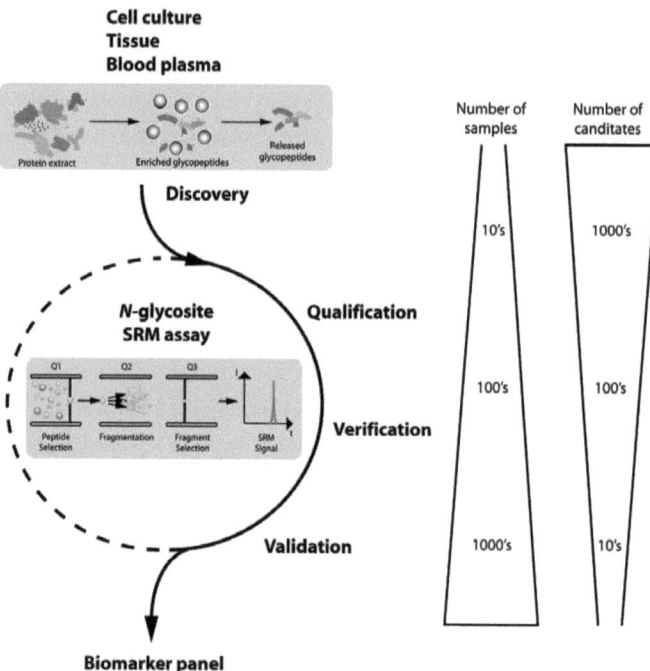

Figure 1.6 Scheme for Biomarker discovery, qualification, verification and validation. Solid phase enrichment of N-glycopeptides (SPEG) can be performed to discover *in vivo* disease specific signatures using cells, tissue and finally blood plasma and MS-based label-free quantification. The selected reaction monitoring (SRM) assays of these proteins are then qualified and later verified in human patients by SRM and eventually validated again by SRM or ELISA.

1 - Introduction

1.6 References

1. Lander, E.S. et al. Initial sequencing and analysis of the human genome. *Nature* **409**, 860-921 (2001).
2. Venter, J.C. et al. The sequence of the human genome. *Science* **291**, 1304-51 (2001).
3. Consortium, I.H.G.S. Finishing the euchromatic sequence of the human genome. *Nature* **431**, 931-45 (2004).
4. Lottspeich, F. Proteome Analysis: A Pathway to the Functional Analysis of Proteins. *Angew Chem Int Ed Engl* **38**, 2476-2492 (1999).
5. Proud, C.G. The eukaryotic initiation factor 4E-binding proteins and apoptosis. *Cell Death Differ* **12**, 541-6 (2005).
6. Tischer, C. & Bastiens, P.I. Lateral phosphorylation propagation: an aspect of feedback signalling? *Nat Rev Mol Cell Biol* **4**, 971-4 (2003).
7. Restle, A., Janz, C. & Wiesmüller, L. Differences in the association of p53 phosphorylated on serine 15 and key enzymes of homologous recombination. *Oncogene* **24**, 4380-7 (2005).
8. Spiriti, J., Bogani, F., van der Vaart, A. & Ghirlanda, G. Modulation of protein stability by O-glycosylation in a designed Gc-MAF analog. *Biophys Chem* **134**, 157-67 (2008).
9. Aebersold, R.H. & Mann, M. Mass spectrometry-based proteomics. *Nature* **422**, 198-207 (2003).
10. Fenn, J.B., Mann, M., Meng, C.K., Wong, S.F. & Whitehouse, C.M. Electrospray ionization for mass spectrometry of large biomolecules. *Science* **246**, 64-71 (1989).
11. Hillenkamp, F., Karas, M., Beavis, R.C. & Chait, B.T. Matrix-assisted laser desorption/ionization mass spectrometry of biopolymers. *Anal Chem* **63**, 1193A-1203A (1991).
12. de Godoy, L.M. et al. Status of complete proteome analysis by mass spectrometry: SILAC labeled yeast as a model system. *Genome Biol* **7**, R50 (2006).
13. Schmidt, A. et al. An integrated, directed mass spectrometric approach for in-depth characterization of complex peptide mixtures. *Mol Cell Proteomics* **7**, 2138-50 (2008).
14. Domon, B. & Aebersold, R.H. Mass spectrometry and protein analysis. *Science* **312**, 212-7 (2006).
15. Hood, L., Heath, J.R., Phelps, M.E. & Lin, B. Systems biology and new technologies enable predictive and preventative medicine. *Science* **306**, 640-3 (2004).
16. Goncalves, A., Borg, J. & Pouyssegur, J. Biomarkers in cancer management: a crucial bridge toward personalized medicine. *Drug Discovery Today: Therapeutic Strategies* **1**, 305-311 (2004).
17. Jain, K.K. Role of oncoproteomics in the personalized management of cancer. *Expert review of proteomics* **1**, 49-55 (2004).
18. van 't Veer, L.J. et al. Gene expression profiling predicts clinical outcome of breast cancer. *Nature* **415**, 530-6 (2002).
19. van de Vijver, M.J. et al. A gene-expression signature as a predictor of survival in breast cancer. *N Engl J Med* **347**, 1999-2009 (2002).
20. Chang, J.C. et al. Gene expression profiling for the prediction of therapeutic response to docetaxel in patients with breast cancer. *Lancet* **362**, 362-9 (2003).
21. Staunton, J.E. et al. Chemosensitivity prediction by transcriptional profiling. *Proc Natl Acad Sci USA* **98**, 10787-92 (2001).
22. Paik, S. et al. A multigene assay to predict recurrence of tamoxifen-treated, node-negative breast cancer. *N Engl J Med* **351**, 2817-26 (2004).
23. Liotta, L.A. & Petricoin, E.F. Serum peptidome for cancer detection: spinning biologic trash into diagnostic gold. *J Clin Invest* **116**, 26-30 (2006).
24. Zhang, H. et al. Mass spectrometric detection of tissue proteins in plasma. *Mol Cell Proteomics* **6**, 64-71 (2007).
25. Rao, A., Motiwala, H.G. & Karim, O.M. The discovery of prostate-specific antigen. *BJU Int* **101**, 5-10 (2008).
26. Flocks, R.H., URICH, V.C., PATEL, C.A. & OPITZ, J.M. Studies on the antigenic properties of prostatic tissue. I. *J Urol* **84**, 134-43 (1960).
27. Hara, M., Koyanagi, Y., Inoue, T. & Fukuyama, T. [Some physico-chemical characteristics of " -seminoprotein", an antigenic component specific for human seminal plasma. Forensic immunological study of body fluids and secretion. VII]. *Nihon Hoigaku Zasshi* **25**, 322-4 (1971).
28. Stamey, T.A. et al. Prostate-specific antigen as a serum marker for adenocarcinoma of the prostate. *N Engl J Med* **317**, 909-16 (1987).
29. Schechter, A.L. et al. The neu oncogene: an erb-B-related gene encoding a 185,000-Mr tumour antigen. *Nature* **312**, 513-6 (1984).
30. Slamon, D.J. et al. Human breast cancer: correlation of relapse and survival with amplification of the HER-2/neu oncogene. *Science* **235**, 177-82 (1987).
31. Luftner, D., Lüke, C. & Possinger, K. Serum HER-2/neu in the management of breast cancer patients. *Clin Biochem* **36**, 233-40 (2003).
32. Baselga, J., Norton, L., Albanell, J., Kim, Y.M. & Mendelsohn, J. Recombinant humanized anti-HER2 antibody (Herceptin) enhances the antitumor activity of paclitaxel and doxorubicin against HER2/neu overexpressing human breast cancer xenografts. *Cancer Res* **58**, 2825-31 (1998).
33. Thompson, I.M. et al. Effect of finasteride on the sensitivity of PSA for detecting prostate cancer. *J Natl Cancer Inst* **98**, 1128-33 (2006).

1.6 References

34. Cook, G.B. et al. Clinical utility of serum HER-2/neu testing on the Bayer Immuno 1 automated system in breast cancer. *Anticancer Res* **21**, 1465-70 (2001).
35. Pritzker, K.P. Cancer biomarkers: easier said than done. *Clin Chem* **48**, 1147-50 (2002).
36. Jones, H. On a New Substance Occurring in the Urine of a Patient with Mollities Ossium. *Philosophical Transactions of the Royal Society of London (1776-1886)* **138**, 55-62 (2006).
37. Kyle, R.A. Multiple myeloma: how did it begin? *Mayo Clin Proc* **69**, 680-3 (1994).
38. Sinclair, D., Dagg, J.H., Smith, J.G. & Stott, D.I. The incidence and possible relevance of Bence-Jones protein in the sera of patients with multiple myeloma. *Br J Haematol* **62**, 689-94 (1986).
39. Srinivas, P.R., Verma, M., Zhao, Y. & Srivastava, S. Proteomics for cancer biomarker discovery. *Clin Chem* **48**, 1160-9 (2002).
40. Lee, S.J. et al. Mannose receptor-mediated regulation of serum glycoprotein homeostasis. *Science* **295**, 1898-901 (2002).
41. Petricoin, E.F. et al. Use of proteomic patterns in serum to identify ovarian cancer. *Lancet* **359**, 572-7 (2002).
42. Zhang, H. et al. High throughput quantitative analysis of serum proteins using glycopeptide capture and liquid chromatography mass spectrometry. *Mol Cell Proteomics* **4**, 144-55 (2005).
43. Hong, S.H. et al. An autoantibody-mediated immune response to calreticulin isoforms in pancreatic cancer. *Cancer Res* **64**, 5504-10 (2004).
44. Radulovic, D. et al. Informatics Platform for Global Proteomic Profiling and Biomarker Discovery Using Liquid Chromatography-Tandem Mass Spectrometry. *Molecular & Cellular Proteomics* **3**, 984 (2004).
45. Janzi, M. et al. Serum Microarrays for Large Scale Screening of Protein Levels *Molecular & Cellular Proteomics* **4**, 1942 (2005).
46. Anderson, N.L. & Anderson, N.G. The human plasma proteome: history, character, and diagnostic prospects. *Mol Cell Proteomics* **1**, 845-67 (2002).
47. States, D.J. et al. Challenges in deriving high-confidence protein identifications from data gathered by a HUPO plasma proteome collaborative study. *Nat Biotechnol* **24**, 333-8 (2006).
48. Polanski, M. & Anderson, N.L. Candidate Cancer Markers. *Biomarker Insights* **2**, 48 (2006).
49. Herrmann, W. et al. The measurement of complexed prostate-specific antigen has a better performance than total prostate-specific antigen. *Clin Chem Lab Med* **42**, 1051-7 (2004).
50. Ng, T.K., Vasilareas, D., Mitterdorfer, A.J., Maher, P.O. & Lalak, A. Prostate cancer detection with digital rectal examination, prostate-specific antigen, transrectal ultrasonography and biopsy in clinical urological practice. *BJU Int* **95**, 545-8 (2005).
51. Wu, J. Circulating Tumor Markers of the New Millennium: Target Therapy, Early Detection, and Prognosis (2002).
52. Echan, L.A., Tang, H.Y., Ali-Khan, N., Lee, K. & Speicher, D.W. Depletion of multiple high-abundance proteins improves protein profiling capacities of human serum and plasma. *Proteomics* **5**, 3292-303 (2005).
53. Brand, J., Haslberger, T., Zolg, W., Pestlin, G. & Palme, S. Depletion efficiency and recovery of trace markers from a multiparameter immunodepletion column. *Proteomics* **6**, 3236-42 (2006).
54. Zolg, W. The proteomic search for diagnostic biomarkers: lost in translation? *Mol Cell Proteomics* **5**, 1720-6 (2006).
55. Domon, B. & Aebersold, R.H. Challenges and opportunities in proteomics data analysis. *Mol Cell Proteomics* **5**, 1921-6 (2006).
56. Rifai, N., Gillette, M.A. & Carr, S.A. Protein biomarker discovery and validation: the long and uncertain path to clinical utility. *Nat Biotechnol* **24**, 971-83 (2006).
57. Altmüller, J., Palmer, L.J., Fischer, G., Scherb, H. & Wjst, M. Genomewide scans of complex human diseases: true linkage is hard to find. *Am J Hum Genet* **69**, 936-50 (2001).
58. Coombes, K.R., Morris, J.S., Hu, J., Edmonson, S.R. & Baggerly, K.A. Serum proteomics profiling--a young technology begins to mature. *Nat Biotechnol* **23**, 291-2 (2005).
59. Nedelkov, D., Kiernan, U.A., Niederkofler, E.E., Tubbs, K.A. & Nelson, R.W. Investigating diversity in human plasma proteins. *Proc Natl Acad Sci U S A* **102**, 10852-7 (2005).
60. Kuick, R. et al. Discovery of cancer biomarkers through the use of mouse models. *Cancer Lett* **249**, 40-8 (2007).
61. Tyers, M. & Mann, M. From genomics to proteomics. *Nature* **422**, 193-7 (2003).
62. Eriksson, J. & Fenyö, D. Improving the success rate of proteome analysis by modeling protein-abundance distributions and experimental designs. *Nat Biotechnol* **25**, 651-5 (2007).
63. Staging: Questions and Answers. *National Cancer Institute Fact Sheet 5.32* (2004).
64. Gleason, D.F. Histologic grading of prostate cancer: a perspective. *Hum Pathol* **23**, 273-9 (1992).
65. Ludwig, J.A. & Weinstein, J.N. Biomarkers in cancer staging, prognosis and treatment selection. *Nat Rev Cancer* **5**, 845-56 (2005).
66. Zhang, H., Li, X.J., Martin, D.B. & Aebersold, R.H. Identification and quantification of N-linked glycoproteins using hydrazide chemistry, stable isotope labeling and mass spectrometry. *Nat Biotechnol* **21**, 660-6 (2003).
67. Gahmberg, C.G. & Tolvanen, M. Why mammalian cell surface proteins are glycoproteins. *Trends Biochem Sci* **21**, 308-11 (1996).
68. Yang, Z. & Hancock, W.S. Approach to the comprehensive analysis of glycoproteins isolated from human serum using a multi-lectin affinity column. *J Chromatogr A* **1053**, 79-88 (2004).

1 - Introduction

69. Bayer, E.A., Ben-Hur, H. & Wilchek, M. Biocytin hydrazide--a selective label for sialic acids, galactose, and other sugars in glycoconjugates using avidin-biotin technology. *Anal Biochem* **170**, 271-81 (1988).
70. Tian, Y., Zhou, Y., Elliott, S., Aebersold, R.H. & Zhang, H. Solid-phase extraction of N-linked glycopeptides. *Nat Protoc* **2**, 334-9 (2007).
71. Wollscheid, B. et al. Mass-spectrometric identification and relative quantification of N-linked cell surface glycoproteins. *Nat Biotechnol* **27**, 378-86 (2009).
72. Yildirim, M.A., Goh, K.I., Cusick, M.E., Barabási, A.L. & Vidal, M. Drug-target network. *Nat Biotechnol* **25**, 1119-26 (2007).
73. Malmstrom, J.A. et al. Large scale glycomapping in human plasma. *manuscript in preparation*.
74. Zhang, H. et al. UniPep--a database for human N-linked glycosites: a resource for biomarker discovery. *Genome Biol* **7**, R73 (2006).
75. Deutsch, E.W. et al. Human Plasma PeptideAtlas. *Proteomics* (2005).
76. Desiere, F. et al. Integration with the human genome of peptide sequences obtained by high-throughput mass spectrometry. *Genome Biol* **6**, R9 (2005).
77. Deutsch, E.W., Lam, H. & Aebersold, R.H. PeptideAtlas: a resource for target selection for emerging targeted proteomics workflows. *EMBO Rep* **9**, 429-34 (2008).
78. Bantscheff, M., Schirle, M., Sweetman, G., Rick, J. & Kuster, B. Quantitative mass spectrometry in proteomics: a critical review. *Analytical and bioanalytical chemistry* **389**, 1017-31 (2007).
79. Mueller, L.N., Brusniak, M.Y., Mani, D.R. & Aebersold, R.H. An Assessment of Software Solutions for the Analysis of Mass Spectrometry Based Quantitative Proteomics Data. *J Proteome Res* **7**, 51-61 (2008).
80. Gygi, S.P. et al. Quantitative analysis of complex protein mixtures using isotope-coded affinity tags. *Nat Biotechnol* **17**, 994-9 (1999).
81. Liu, H., Sadygov, R.G. & Yates, J.R. A model for random sampling and estimation of relative protein abundance in shotgun proteomics. *Anal Chem* **76**, 4193-201 (2004).
82. Ishihama, Y. et al. Exponentially modified protein abundance index (emPAI) for estimation of absolute protein amount in proteomics by the number of sequenced peptides per protein. *Mol Cell Proteomics* **4**, 1265-72 (2005).
83. Listgarten, J. & Emili, A. Statistical and computational methods for comparative proteomic profiling using liquid chromatography-tandem mass spectrometry. *Mol Cell Proteomics* **4**, 419-34 (2005).
84. Mueller, L.N. et al. SuperHirn - a novel tool for high resolution LC-MS-based peptide/protein profiling. *Proteomics* **7**, 3470-80 (2007).
85. Schiess, R. et al. Analysis of cell surface proteome changes via label-free, quantitative proteomics. *Mol Cell Proteomics* **8**, 624-38 (2009).
86. Mallick, P. et al. Computational prediction of proteotypic peptides for quantitative proteomics. *Nat Biotechnol* **25**, 125-31 (2007).
87. Kuster, B., Schirle, M., Mallick, P. & Aebersold, R.H. Scoring proteomes with proteotypic peptide probes. *Nat Rev Mol Cell Biol* **6**, 577-83 (2005).
88. Tang, H. et al. A computational approach toward label-free protein quantification using predicted peptide detectability. *Bioinformatics* **22**, e481-8 (2006).
89. Kuhn, E. et al. Quantification of C-reactive protein in the serum of patients with rheumatoid arthritis using multiple reaction monitoring mass spectrometry and 13C-labeled peptide standards. *Proteomics* **4**, 1175-86 (2004).
90. Stahl-Zeng, J. et al. High sensitivity detection of plasma proteins by multiple reaction monitoring of N-glycosites. *Mol Cell Proteomics* **6**, 1809-17 (2007).
91. Lange, V. et al. Targeted quantitative analysis of Streptococcus pyogenes virulence factors by multiple reaction monitoring. *Mol Cell Proteomics* **7**, 1489-500 (2008).

2 Selective isolation and MS-based identification of O-linked glycopeptides

2.1 Authorship

The strategy presented here was specifically developed for the identification of formerly O-linked glycopeptides (O-glycosites) as an addition to the previously established method in our lab for N-glycosites. A manuscript describing the proteomic O-glycosite identification strategy including its application is currently in preparation. I developed the main ideas and concept of this strategy and performed the initial data analysis. I would like to gratefully acknowledge Reto Wijker who worked together with me on this project during his Semesterwork and Masterthesis. He performed the O-glycosite strategy optimization experiments with respect to the specific reaction conditions and the test experiments. Without his contributions, this work would not have been accomplished. James Sorell Eddes was very critical in implementing modifications in the bioinformatic processing pipeline of O-glycosite identification. Furthermore I would like to thank Alexander Schmidt, Bernd Wollscheid, and Bruno Domon for helpful discussions. The project was performed under the supervision of Ruedi Aebersold.

2.2 Summary

Discovery-driven protein identification using mass-spectrometry (MS) is still hampered by the extreme dynamic range of protein concentrations in complex biological samples. Typically, a few highly expressed protein species, such as human serum albumin in blood or ribosomal proteins in the cytosol, dominate such samples and limit the identification of lower abundant proteins in today's MS-based protein identification strategies. Therefore, there is a strong need for technologies which enable the identification of low abundant proteins and specific subproteomes such post-translationally modified proteins. The recent development of targeted mass spectrometry-based strategies has enabled researchers to analyze proteins at very low concentrations. In addition to depletion of high abundant proteins or multidimensional protein fractionation, the enrichment of certain subproteomes such as the phospho-proteome, and the glyco-proteome has proven to be successful. Specifically, the glyco-proteome enrichment strategy focuses on a very relevant subproteome in the context of diagnostic research, since these proteins are mainly present on the cell surface and secreted into the body fluids such as blood. The current protocol for solid phase extracted glycoproteins focuses only on the N-glycosites, while O-glycosites are neglected due to the lack of an appropriate isolation strategy. We have established a novel strategy that allows not only for the identification of N-, but also for O-glycosites using a chemical approach. The strategy and results presented here show that O-glycosites can now be identified in a multiplexed and unbiased fashion using proteomic technology.

2.3 Introduction

In the past, mass-spectrometry based proteomics has proven to be a powerful tool[1]. Recent improvements in both the instrumental setup and the upfront processing of biological samples has enabled researchers to map out the majority of the proteome of selected organisms[2, 3]. However, certain proteomes such as body fluids still remain largely uncovered due mainly to two reasons; firstly, the extreme dynamic range of protein concentration, as in the case of blood is expected to be in the range of 10 to 12 orders of magnitude; secondly, such proteomes are often dominated by a few extraordinarily highly abundant proteins. For example, human serum albumin represents more than 50% of the total protein mass in human plasma. Furthermore, 90% of the plasma protein mass is constituted by only 10 different protein species and the 22 most abundant plasma proteins comprise 99% of this proteome. This is evident in typical shotgun experiments where highly abundant proteins are repeatedly sequenced and that lower abundance protein signals are suppressed by their dominating counterparts.

In order to circumvent this problem, three main approaches are typically employed. High abundant proteins can be depleted from the sample using affinity based protein depletion columns. Up to 20 proteins can be efficiently depleted using commercially available columns[4]. Multidimensional protein separation using gel-based approaches such as 2D-gel electrophoresis or free-flow electrophoresis and strong cation exchange-chromatography in combination with online reversed-phase HPLC peptide separation coupled to MS have proven to be successful[5]. Lastly, the enrichment of subproteomes is an attractive alternative to the approaches just mentioned in order to lower sample complexity. Thereby the chemical properties of certain rarely occurring amino acids such as cysteine[6] or protein modifications such as phosphorylation[7] or glycosylation[8] can be used to selectively enrich these proteomes. Focusing on a specific subset of proteins not only reduces sample complexity, but also offers the possibility to target subproteomes implicated in specific biological functions. Such strategies were implemented very successfully, for example, in the activity-based profiling of phosphatases[9], or the identification of phosphorylation sites[10]. The development and application of such strategies now enables the study of dynamic signaling events over time in biological systems.

We have focused our research on glycoproteins which are an ideal subproteome to target as they are known to be present selectively on the cell surface or destined for secretion[11]. While cell surface proteins represent ideal diagnostic and therapeutic targets, secreted proteins can be easily detected in body fluids

2 - Selective isolation and MS-based identification of O-linked glycopeptides

and thus can be used as diagnostic markers for remote sensing of disease. We have developed a method for the analysis of N-linked glycoproteins and the identification of N-linked glycosites[8]. We have also shown that focus on glycosites significantly increases the analytical depth compared to whole serum analysis[12] as the selective enrichment of glycosites significantly reduces the complexity of the sample. We have furthermore shown high-speed proteome screening methods can be based on the selective, mass spectrometric analysis of glycosites[13]. However, current protocols for the identification of glycopeptides are limited to the identification of N-glycosites. While N-linked glycopeptides immobilized on a hydrazide-based solid surface can be readily isolated through the selective release of the glycans by PNGase F, O-linked glycopeptides are more difficult to study for an unavailability of an enzyme that reliably removes immobilized O-linked glycans. Nevertheless, current N-glycosite enrichment-based efforts would greatly profit from an expansion to O-glycosites in order to achieve a more complete coverage of the glyco-subproteome and thus a strategy to isolate both types of glycosites is needed.

Global analysis of O-glycosylation still remains a challenging analytical problem. O-glycan structures vary considerably; there is no consensus-motif for O-glycosylation, and there is no known endo-acting enzyme that is generally applicable for the removal of O-linked glycans. The most commonly used enzyme is O-glycanase (Endo-β-N-acetylgalactosaminidase) that displays strict substrate specificity and removes the entire glycan only if the disaccharide galactosyl-β-1-3-GalNAc is attached to serine or threonine. In a recent study Hägglund et al. presented an enzymatic deglycosylation scheme enabling the identification of N- and O-glycosylation site mapping. While N-glycosylation sites could be reliably identified in this study, the enzyme–based identification of O-glycosylation sites was hampered by the fact that O-linked glycans, in general, are structurally more diverse than N-glycans and that for global trimming a complex exoglycosidase cocktail is needed[14]. Additionally, through the solid phase enrichment of glycoproteins, cis-diol containing carbohydrate moieties are modified by periodate oxidation and thus mostly resistant to enzymatic treatment. Chemical removal of glycans can be achieved by trifluoromethanesulphonic acid[15] or by β-elimination under alkaline conditions [16, 17]. A drawback with the β-elimination reaction is the low specificity, since both phosphorylated and, to a lesser extent, unmodified serine and threonine residues also may be modified in β-elimination. Given these current limitations, O-glycosylation analysis poses a so far unsolved problem.

Here we describe a strategy for the consecutive release of N- and O-glycosites from a solid support enabling specific enrichment for the purpose of subsequent MS identification. In contrast to the enzymatic deglycosylation of N-linked glycoproteins by PNGase F, we utilized a chemical approach for the release of O-linked glycans previously described by Rusnak et al.[18]. To achieve high reproducibility and specificity, we used a synthetic O-linked glycopeptide for the optimization of the glycan release by alkaline β-elimination and the subsequent Michael addition of cysteamine (CA) to the formerly glycosylated serine or threonine residue to unambiguously identify O-glycosylation sites. Additionally, the addition of CA to serines or threonines introduces a new trypsin cleavage site that can be used as a secondary filter and thus increases the certainty of new identifications. We then combined the selective enrichment of glycoproteins with the specific release of O-glycosites from the solid-phase employing a model glycoprotein. Finally, we show the combined identification of both N- and O-glycosites in blood serum.

2.4 Experimental Procedures

Chemicals. Porcine trypsin, modified, sequencing grade, was purchased from Promega (Madison, WI, USA). Tris(2-carboxyethyl)phosphine (TCEP), iodoacetamide and α-cyano-4-hydroxycinnamic acid were purchased from Fluka (Buchs, Switzerland). HPLC-grade water and acetonitrile were purchased from Riedel-de Haën (Seelze, Germany), sodium periodate (Perbio, Switzerland), 15 ml Dounce Tissue Grinder (Wheaton, USA), RapiGest (Waters), PNGase F (NEB), Affi-Prep Hz Hydrazide (BioRad). The synthetic glycopeptide (CTD-peptide) was a gift from Gerald W. Hart from Johns Hopkins University, Baltimore, USA. Blood serum from a single male donor was obtained from Blutspende Zürich, Switzerland.

Immobilization of glycopeptides on hydrazide resin. Glycoproteins were enriched from cell culture using the protocol published by H. Zhang et al.[8]. Glycoproteins in coupling buffer (0.1 M sodium acetate and 150 mM NaCl, pH 5.5) were oxidized by adding 15 mM of sodium periodate at room temperature for 1 h. After removal of sodium periodate, the sample was conjugated to the hydrazide resin at room temperature for 10-24 h. Non-glycoproteins were then removed by washing the resin 6 times with an equal amount of urea solution (8 M urea/0.2 M NH_4HCO_3/0.05% (w/v) SDS/ 5 mM EDTA, pH 8.3). After the last wash and the removal of urea solution, the resin was diluted with 3 bed volumes of water. Trypsin was added at a ratio of 1 μg of trypsin to 200 μg of protein and digested at 37°C overnight. The resulting peptides were reduced by adding 5 mM TCEP at 37°C for 30 min, and alkylated using 10 mM iodoacetamide for 30 min at room temperature. The trypsin released peptides were removed by washing the resin 10x with 1.5 M NaCl, pure methanol, 80% (v/v) acetonitrile, 50 mM NH_4HCO_3.

Dephosphorylation. The peptides and proteins were treated with both shrimp alkaline phosphatase (SAP) and calf intestine phosphatase (CIP) to remove the phosphate groups from the phosphorylation sites. Since serine and threonines undergo alkaline β-elimination if they are either glycosylated or phosphorylated, dephosphorylation is first necessary to enable unambiguous identifications of O-linked

2 - Selective isolation and MS-based identification of O-linked glycopeptides

glycosylation sites. Dried samples were resolved in 1x NEBuffer 3 and incubated with 5 U of each of CIP and SAP for 2-4 h on a shaker (1'000 rpm) at 37°C. The enzymatic reaction was stopped by heating the samples for 15 min at 85°C.

Release of N-linked glycopeptides from hydrazide resin. The enzyme PNGase F was used to remove N-linked glycopeptides from the solid phase. The hydrazide beads with the bound peptides were washed 10x with 500 µl 100 mM NH_4HCO_3 pH 7.8. Then 1 µl of PNGase F was added to 1 µl 100 mM of NH_4HCO_3 pH 7.8 and 50 ml of this solution was added to 50 µl of dry beads. The samples were incubated on a shaker (1000 rpm) at 37°C overnight. Then they were centrifuged and the flow-through was collected. After this, the beads were washed twice with 80% acetonitrile/ddH$_2$O and the flow-through was collected as well. Released N-glycosites were dried in a speed vac concentrator and re-solubilized in 0.1% formic acid for mass spectrometric analysis.

Release of O-linked glycopeptides from hydrazide resin by β-elimination and Michael addition of cysteamine. Glycopeptides were released from the hydrazide support by adding $Ba(OH)_2$ at pH 11.6 with 0.2 M CA to the beads and incubated for 24 h at 40°C on a shaker (1'000 rpm) under argon. The samples were then acidified with formic acid to stop the reaction. Released O-glycosites were dried in a speed vac concentrator and re-solubilized in 0.1% formic acid for mass spectrometric analysis.

Matrix-assisted laser desorption/ionization mass spectrometry. A matrix-assisted laser desorption/ionisation (MALDI) combined with a tandem time-of-flight MS/MS system (4800 *Plus* MALDI-TOF/TOF™ Analyzer from ABI) was used to evaluate and optimize the β-elimination, Michael addition with CA and enrichment methods with the model glycopeptide. The dried samples were resuspended in 50% acetonitrile and 0.1% trifluoroacetic acid. 1 µL containing 0.5 nmol of the peptide solution was spotted together with 1 µL of 10 mg/ml α-cyano-4-hydroxycinnamic acid (matrix) on a MALDI plate. The spots were dried and analyzed by the 4800 Plus MALDI-TOF/TOF™ Analyzer.

Electrospray ionization mass spectrometry. Samples were analyzed on a LTQ mass spectrometer (Thermo Electron, San Jose, CA) equipped with a nanoelectrospray ion source. Chromatographic separation of peptides was performed on an Agilent 1100 micro HPLC system (Waldbronn, Germany), equipped with a 10 cm fused silica emitter, 150 µm inner diameter, packed with a Magic C18 AQ 5 µm resin (Michrom BioResources, Auburn, CA, USA). Peptides were loaded on the column using a cooled (8°C) Agilent autosampler and separated with a linear gradient of 5 to 40% acetonitrile containing 0.1% formic acid over 55 min at a flow rate of 5.8 µl/min. For each peptide sample, a standard data-dependent acquisition (DDA) where the three most intense ions per MS-scan are selected for CID was performed. A threshold of 3'000 ion counts was set to trigger an MS/MS attempt.

2.4 Experimental Procedures

Data analysis. Data acquired by the MALDI-TOF/TOF instrument was analyzed using the GPS Explorer software (ABI) v4.9. The raw data acquired by the LTQ mass spectrometer (software: Xcalibur 2.0 SR1) was converted to mzXML using ReAdW 3.5.1[19] applying default parameters. MS/MS scans were then exported as .dta files without further processing using the program mzXML2Other[19]. MS/MS spectra acquired form the model protein Fetuin-A were searched against the NCBI Haemophilus influenzae Rd database (1787 entries) containing the bovine Fetuin-A sequence using SEQUEST v.27[20]. The five known O-linked glycosylation sites in bovine Fetuin-A, Ser-253, Thr-262, Ser-264, Ser-278 and Ser-323 were all exchanged with a lysine. The SEQUEST database search criteria included static modifications of 57 Da for cysteines (for the alkylation with iodoacetamide) and specifically for the O-glycosite containing sample variable modifications for lysine of 18 Da and 32 Da for CA modified serines and threonines, respectively. In this way, a tryptic search constraint could be applied. For the N-glycosite sample, a variable modification of 1 Da for potential formerly N-glycosylated asparagines (which are converted to aspartic acid by PNGase F release) was used instead of the lysine modifications. The following additional search constraints were applied: average parent and fragment masses, precursor-ion mass tolerance: 2 Da, fragment-ion mass tolerance 0.5 Da, 1 missed cleavage. The identified N-and O-glycosites were processed and analyzed through the mass spectrometry Trans-Proteomic Pipeline 3.5 (TPP)[21]. ProteinProphet allowed filtering of large-scale data sets with assessment of predictable sensitivity and false positive identification error rates. In this study, we used a PeptideProphet probability score threshold of ≥ 0.9.

MS/MS spectra obtained from the blood serum analysis were searched against the International Protein Index (IPI) human protein database (version 3.38) using SEQUEST. The SEQUEST database search criteria included static modifications of 57 Da for cysteines (for the alkylation with iodoacetamide) and variable modifications of either 1 Da for potential formerly N-glycosylated asparagines (which are converted to aspartic acid by PNGase F release) or 59 for potential formerly O-glycosylated serines and threonines (which are modified by CA), respectively. The database search results for the N-glycosite containing sample were evaluated by PeptideProphet as described above. In the case of O-glycosites, instead of using PeptideProphet, we used the following SEQUEST score cutoffs: Xcorr > 2.5, ΔC_n > 0.1, and SpRank < 5 (applied to all peptide charge states). 1. The cross-correlation (Xcorr) is a measure based on the number of peaks of common mass between observed and expected spectra, and used as a primary criterion for peptide assignments; 2. ΔC_n is the relative difference between the first and second highest Xcorr score for all peptides queried from the database; 3. SpRank is a measure of how well the assigned peptide scored relative to those of similar mass in the database, using a preliminary correlation metric.

2 - Selective Isolation and MS-based Identification of O-linked Glycopeptides

2.5 Results

The goal of this project was to develop a fast and reproducible strategy for the multiplexed identification of O-glycosites. Therefore we first established the reaction conditions for the release of O-linked glycans from glycopeptides using a model O-linked glycopeptide. We then combined the selective enrichment of glycoproteins with the specific isolation of O-glycosites by releasing the peptide from its solid-phase captured O-linked glycan moieties using a model glycoprotein. Finally, we applied the technology to blood serum.

2.5.1 Specific glycan release and site mapping of O-glycosylation

To release O-linked glycan from the peptide we used β-elimination of glycoserine residues to generate dehydroalanine under basic conditions (glycothreonine is converted to β-methyldehydroalanine). Similar chemistry has been used to enrich and quantify phosphoproteins for traditional trypsin digestion and MS/MS sequencing[22-27]. In the next step, dehydroalanine acts as a Michael acceptor for CA, generating an aminoethylcysteine residue (for glycothreonine, β-methylaminoethylcysteine is generated) (Figure 2.1). Because aminoethylcysteine is isosteric with lysine, proteases that recognize lysine (e.g., trypsin, Lys-C and lysyl endopeptidase) will cleave proteins at this residue. The same strategy has been successfully used for phosphopeptide site mapping[28].

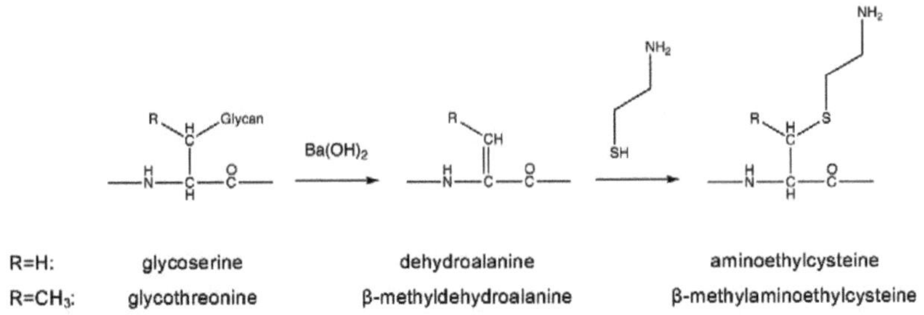

R=H: glycoserine   dehydroalanine   aminoethylcysteine
R=CH$_3$: glycothreonine   β-methyldehydroalanine   β-methylaminoethylcysteine

Figure 2.1 Scheme for transformation of glycoserine/ glycothreonine residue to dehdroalanine/ β-methyl-Dehydroalanine via β-elimination and then to aminoethylcysteine/ β-methylaminoethylcysteine by Michael-addition of cystamine.

The introduction of an additional trypsin cleavage site is a critical point of the strategy presented here. It adds a second layer of certainty by having a specific cleavage site in addition to the modified amino acid residue and thus increases the specificity for the unambiguous assignment of *O*-glycosylation sites. This is an important feature since a common problem with *O*-glycosylation site annotation is the frequent clustering of potential sites in the peptide sequences.

To show the feasibility of the approach, we optimized in a first step the β-elimination reaction of the carbohydrate moieties and the Michael addition of CA. The goal was to get both high yield of the deglycosylated form of the glycopeptides and the highest possible specificity by minimizing side reactions. Furthermore, a good reproducibility should be achieved in order to apply the reaction to complex glycoprotein samples. For this reason a synthetic glycopeptide bearing a tandem repeat of the RNA polymerase II carboxyl terminal domain (CTD) was employed[29]. The repeat sequence YSPTS*PSK (CTD-peptide) contains an *O*-GlcNAc attached at the AA residue Ser-5.

Ammonium hydroxide (NH_4OH), sodium hydroxide (NaOH) and barium hydroxide ($Ba(OH)_2$) have been previously reported to be used successfully for alkaline β-elimination of glycopeptides[18, 30, 31]. Thus the β-elimination combined with the Michael addition of CA was tested with different concentrations of these bases. Additional parameters varied included temperature, incubation time and adduct (CA) concentration. The reaction was found to reach an optimum in respect to the ratio of product (925 *m/z*) to educt (1069 *m/z*) when using $Ba(OH)_2$ at pH 11.35 at 40°C in combination with 200 mM CA for 24 h. The MS spectrum showed both high signal intensity and high specificity for the expected product. Only one minor side reaction occurred which resulted from the unspecific loss of water at a serine or threonine in the absence of any glycosylation and thus the duplicate addition of CA (984 *m/z*). The result was satisfying yielding an educt to product ratio of over 100 although the peak of the intermediate containing the dehydroalanine was still present (Figure 2.2).

Figure 2.2 shows the time dependent release of the carbohydrate moiety by β-elimination forming an intermediate (848 *m/z*) followed by the addition of CA converting it into the final product. An increase of the CA modified peptide could be clearly observed over time indicating an ongoing conversion to the product justifying the long incubation time. Each of the serines and also the threonines present in the model peptide could potentially undergo β-elimination through the loss of water and additional Michael-addition of CA.

2 - Selective isolation and MS-based identification of O-linked glycopeptides

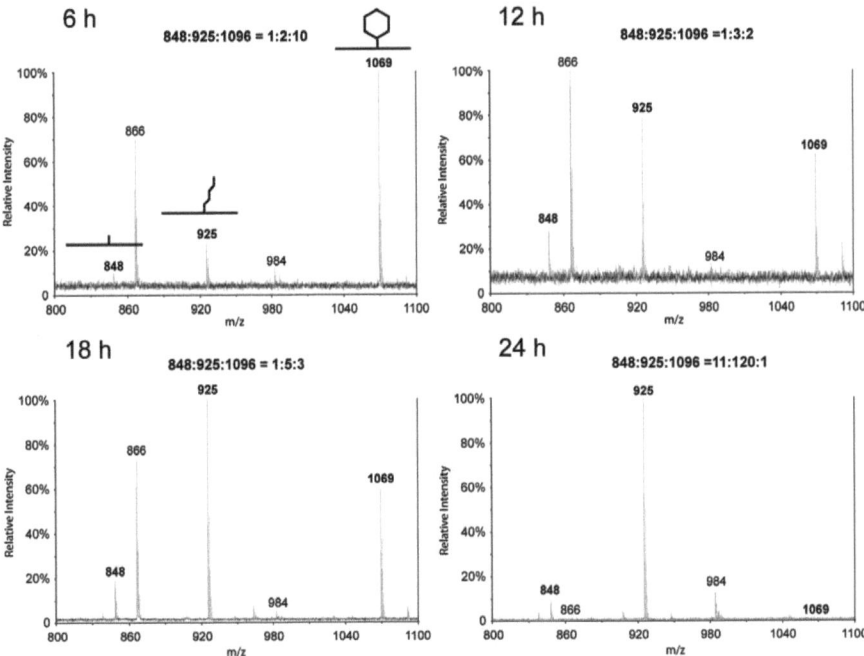

Figure 2.2 Time-dependent conversion of the glycoserine containing glycopeptide (1069 m/z) to the deglycosylated intermediate (848 m/z) and finally to the CA-modified peptide (925 m/z). Shown are the spectra acquired of the same sample after 6, 12, 18, and 24 h respectively.

The MS/MS spectrum shown in Figure 2.3 confirmed that the CA modification occurred exclusively at Ser-5 which was known to be formerly O-glycosylated. No other peaks were detected in the MS/MS spectrum which would indicated another CA position than the expected one. Therefore the applied reaction conditions indicate an optimum in respect to both yield and specificity.

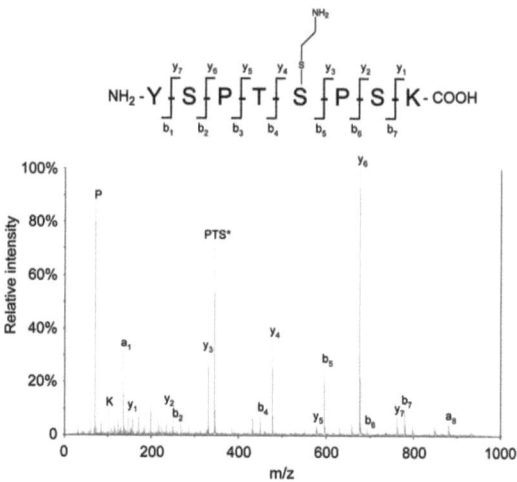

Figure 2.3 MS/MS spectrum of CA-modified CTD-Peptide unambiguously assigned the former site of GlcNAc modification to Ser-5.

2.5.2 Phosphatase treatment to distinguish O-glycosylation and phosphorylation

Phosphoserines and phosphothreonines are modified by β-elimination and Michael-addition of CA just as O-glycosylation sites are[28]. Consequently, it is not possible to distinguish between phosphorylation and O-linked glycosylation sited using the approach as described. However, we tested if phosphatase treatment prior to the β-elimination and Michael addition of CA prevents phosphorylation sites to undergo the modification. To test our hypothesis, the monophosphopeptide FQpSEEQQQTEDELQDK from bovine β-casein (P02666) was mixed with the CTD-peptide.

First, the peptide mixture was treated with phosphatase to reveal if the phosphate group was successfully removed from the monophosphopeptide. The corresponding MS spectra indeed showed the expected mass shift of 80 Da the monophosphopeptide indicating the loss of the phosphate group (Figure 2.4b). Importantly, the dephosphorylation was complete and thus no phosphorylated peptide was present after the treatment which potentially could still undergo modification and lead to a false positive identification of an O-glycosylation site.

Second, β-elimination and Michael-addition of CA were applied to the peptide mixture as without prior phosphatase treatment. The MS spectrum in Figure 2.4c clearly shows that the CA modification was

2 - Selective isolation and MS-based identification of O-linked glycopeptides

incorporated into both the CTD-Peptide as well as the monophosphopeptide (2042 m/z). Therefore no distinction between a phosphorylation and an O-glycosylation site would be possible as expected.

In a third experiment, the peptide sample was dephosphorylated using the phosphatase cocktail followed by β-elimination and Michael addition of CA. Thus only the CTD-peptide should get CA-modified while the dephosphorylated form of the phosphopeptide was expected to not undergo any modification. Our expectations were clearly confirmed by the MS spectrum acquired shown in Figure 2.4d. The minor peak of a CA-modified species originated from the β-elimination product of the phosphopeptide (1965 m/z) already present in the original sample. Here we demonstrated that the application of phosphatases enabled us to rule out the misleading identification of possible phosphorylation sites.

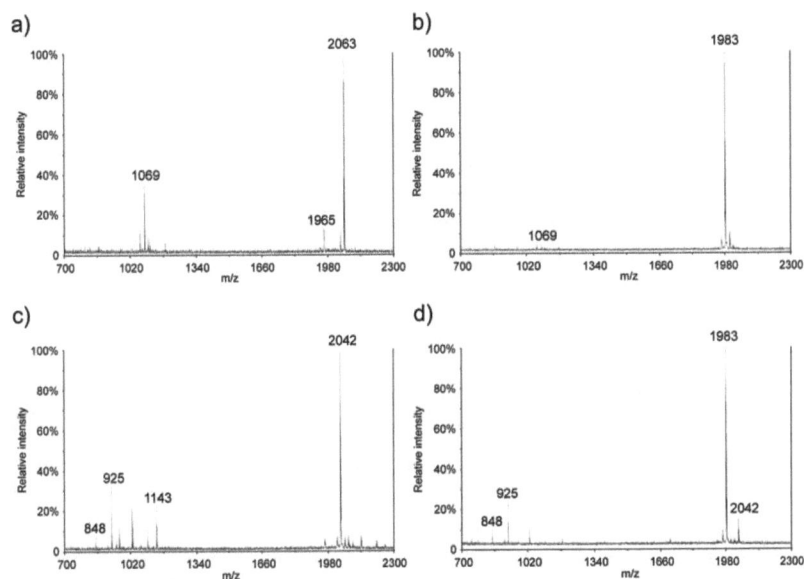

Figure 2.4 a) MS spectrum of the CTD-peptide (1069 m/z) and the monophosphopeptide (2063 m/z). **b)** A loss of 80 m/z of the monophosphopeptide indicated complete dephosphorylation after 4 h of phosphatase treatment. **c)** After β-elimination and Michael addition of CA, both the formerly O-glycosylated CTD-peptide (925 m/z) and the phosphorylated peptide (2042 m/z) reacted alike. **d)** Prior phosphatase treatment allows for the differentiation of glyco- and phosphopeptides because only substituted serines and threonines undergo the chemical conversion.

2.5.3 Selective identification of N- and O-linked glycosites

We have developed an isolation protocol for peptides that contain O-linked carbohydrates that is equivalent for the method developed for the isolation of N-linked glycopeptides termed SPEG (Solid Phase Extraction of Glycopeptides) described by Zhang et al.[8]. The methods share many of the technical elements and steps, including solid-phase capture of glycoproteins out of complex mixtures, analysis of the recovered peptide mixtures by LC-MS/MS and the suite of informatics tools. Importantly, both peptides containing N-linked and O-linked carbohydrates are isolated independently from the same immobilized sample (Figure 2.5).

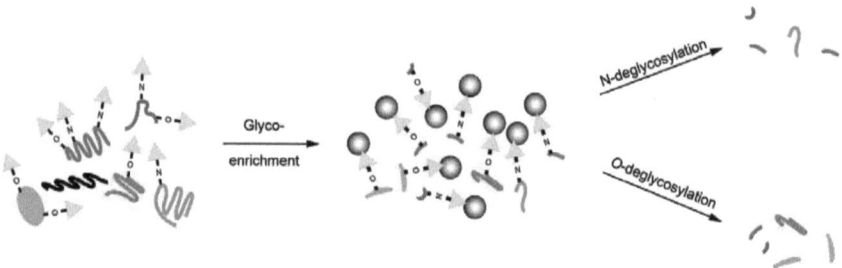

Figure 2.5 Schema for the enrichment of N- and O-glycosites. Glycosylated proteins were enriched on a solid surface followed by trypsinization. After removal of non-glycopeptides, N-linked and O-linked glycopeptides are released separately and ready for LC-MS/MS analysis.

The two methods differ significantly in the recovery of the respective glycopeptides from the solid phase. While N-glycosites can be easily removed by the enzyme called PNGase F, there is no known single enzyme comparable for the release of O-linked glycans. That is why we used the chemical approach which was optimized with the CTD-peptide demonstrated before. Additionally, chemically released O-glycosites were further digested with Lys-C that cleaves CA-modified serines and threonines.

The glycoprotein Alpha-2-HS-glycoprotein (Fetuin-A) from bos taurus containing three N-glycosylation sites, four known O-glycoserines and one O-glycothreonine was chosen to demonstrate the feasibility of this approach[32]. Fetuin-A is a serum protein mediating the transport and availability of a wide variety of cargo substances. The *in silico* digestion of Fetuin-A results in three N-glycopeptides bearing the N-glycosylation sites at Asn-81, Asn-138, and Asn-158. The four O-glycosylation sites at Ser-253, Thr-262, Ser-264, and Ser-278 are all present in one O-glycopeptide, while the fifth, Ser-323, is contained in an additional fully tryptic peptide (Figure 2.6).

2 - Selective Isolation and MS-Based Identification of O-linked Glycopeptides 37

We enriched the glycoprotein on hydrazide beads, digested the protein, and washed away non-glycopeptides. We then first released the N-glycosites and analyzed them by LC-MS/MS. The subsequent database search led to the identification of all three N-glycosites, which confirmed that Fetuin-A was successfully enriched on the solid surface. In a next step we then applied the chemical method in order to release the O-glycosites. The fully tryptic O-glycopeptide, Val^{228}-Arg^{288}, which contains four O-glycosylation sites, would be almost impossible to detect by conventional shot-gun proteomics due to its sequence length of 61 amino acids. In order to overcome this problem, we used the protease Lys-C after the release of O-glycosites from the solid surface. Thereby formerly O-glycosylated serine and threonine residues that were modified by CA were specifically cleaved due to their isosteric characteristic to lysine.

```
        10         20         30         40         50         60
IPLDPVAGYK EPACDDPDTE QAALAAVDYI NKHLPRGYKH TLNQIDSVKV WPRRPTGEVY

        70         80         90        100        110        120
DIEIDTLETT CHVLDPTPLA NCSVRQQTQH AVEGDCDIHV LKQDGQFSVL FTKCDSSPDS

       130        140        150        160        170        180
AEDVRKLCPD CPLLAPLNDS RVVHAVEVAL ATFNAESNGS YLQLVEISRA QFVPLPVSVS

       190        200        210        220        230        240
VEFAVAATDC IAKEVVDPTK CNLLAEKQYG FCKGSVIQKA LGGEDVRVTC TLFQTQPVIP

       250        260        270        280        290        300
QPQPDGAEAE APSAVPDAAG PTPSAAGPPV ASVVVGPSVV AVPLPLHRAH YDLRHTFSGV

       310        320        330        340
ASVESSSGEA FHVGKTPIVG QPSIPGGPVR LCPGRIRYFKI
```

Figure 2.6 Amino acid (AA) sequence of bovine Fetuin-A containing three N-glycosites and two O-glycosites (underlined). N- and O-glycosylation sites are shown in bold.

In order to facilitate a tryptic database search including specific cleavage after modified serine and threonine residues, we changed the known O-glycosylated serine and threonine residues to lysines and allowed mass increments for lysines of 18 and 32 Da. Six fully tryptic peptides of FETUIN-A could be identified using the SEQUEST search software[20]. The O-linked glycopeptide VTCTLFQTQPVIPQPQPDGAEAEAPS* was specifically cut after the modified glycoserine (Ser-253), which indicates that it was formerly glycosylated. Another peptide identified AVPDAAGPT*PS* resulted from the cleavage site of the modified Ser-253 and Ser-264. This again indicates that Ser-253 and Ser-264 were formerly glycosylated. However, the glycosylation site at Thr-262 was solely confirmed by the measurement of an additional mass increment of 59 Da due to the CA modification that occurred upon the release of the *O*-glycan. No specific cleavage was observed after Thr-262. This is because restrictions to the specificity of Lys-C occur when proline is at the carboxylic side of lysine or arginine; the bond is almost completely resistant to cleavage by Lys-C[33]. The two peptides AAGPPVASVVVGPS* and VVAVPLPLHR resulted from the cleavage sites of the modified Ser-264 and Ser-278. The glycosylation site at Ser-323 was confirmed by the identification of the peptide TPIVGQPS*IPGGPVR containing a modified serine with a mass increment of 59 Da corresponding to aminoethylcysteine and additionally by the peptide TPIVGQPS* bearing a specific cleavage site at Ser-323. These data indicate that the two-step conferring specificity provide sufficient selectivity to isolate *O*-glycosites from complex mixtures.

2.5.4 Concurrent identification of *N*- and *O*-glycosites in human serum samples

The final goal was to use the newly developed method for the identification of *O*-glycosites in combination with the well-established selective enrichment of *N*-glycosites from complex samples. Therefore we tested its application to blood serum. To remove high abundant non-glycoproteins, the glycopeptides were enriched using the SPEG method as described before. The immobilized glycoproteins were dephosphorylated so that later no phosphorylation site will be modified by the chemical release strategy for *O*-glycopeptides. After trypsinization and removal of non-glycopeptides, first the *N*-glycopeptides were released with the enzyme PNGase F to test if the method of solid phase extraction of glycopeptides was really successful. The same conditions for β-elimination and Michael addition of CA as established with the CTD-peptide and tested with Fetuin-A were used for the specific release of the *O*-glycopeptides. Then, the *O*-glycopeptides were digested with Lys-C in order to cleave specifically CA-modified serines and threonines.

The mass spectrometric analysis of the sample where *N*-glycopeptides were selectively released with PNGase F from the hydrazide support led to the identification of 400 distinct peptides including 353 peptides containing the *N*-glycosylation motif indicating that they were formerly *N*-glycosylated at a PeptideProphet probability[34] threshold of ≥ 0.9 (FDR 1%). The specificity of almost 90% for *N*-glycosites indicated that the glycoproteins were successfully enriched. The same LC-MS/MS analysis was performed on the *O*-glycosites as described for *N*-glycosites. In contrast to the data analysis of *N*-glycosites, *O*-glycosites could not be processed through the conventional data analysis pipeline. Neither for SEQUEST nor for the TPP an option for the specific cleavage of CA-modified serines and threonines was available. If the same database search parameters as for *N*-glycosites were used, *O*-glycosite identifications got clearly punished for fewer or no tryptic termini. Thus we decided to perform the database search without any restriction to enzyme and instead of calculating the peptide probabilities by PeptideProphet, we used cutoffs of the scores that were obtained by the database search by SEQUEST,

2 - Selective isolation and MS-based identification of O-linked glycopeptides 39

i.e. Xcorr > 2.5, ΔC_n > 0.1, and SpRank < 5 (see method section). Applying these stringent selection criteria resulted in the identification of 95 peptides of which 58 peptides (61%) contained at least one modified serine or threonine (56%) or a serine or threonine precedes the peptide sequence and thus the peptide has a tryptic N-terminus (5%). The same analysis using the identical SEQUEST score cutoffs was done for the N-glycosite analysis. This resulted in the identification of 429 distinct peptides of which 337 were bona fide N-glycosites.

In this experiment we identified 50 O-linked glycoproteins and 88 N-linked glycoproteins (see Supplementary Table S2.1). The four proteins Hemopexin (Beta-1B-glycoprotein), plasma protease C1 inhibitor (C1-inhibiting factor), Alpha-2-HS-glycoprotein precursor (Fetuin-A), and Alpha-1-anti-chymotrypsin precursor (ACT) were identified by both O- and N-glycosites. Among the identified O-glycoproteins are 9 mucins, a family of large, heavily glycosylated proteins known to be O-glycosylated[35]. Furthermore, 13 (26%) of the identified O-glycoproteins were already present in UniPep, a repository for N-glycoproteins and thus experimentally verified glycoproteins. A complete list of the identified O-linked glycoproteins including their site of modification can be found in the Supplementary Table S2.2. We found several O-glycosylation sites previously described such as for the Apolipoprotein C-III (P02760). It is a secreted serum protein predominantly synthesized in liver and to a lesser degree in intestine. The peptide K.FSEFWDLDPEVRPT*SAVAA.- (Figure 2.7a) with the uncleaved CA-modified Thr-74 could verify the O-glycosylation site at Thr-74 as described by Brewer et al.[36].

CA-modified threonines were previously described to be cleaved at these residues less efficiently than compared to CA-modified serines [28]. This could be explained by the steric hindrance of the additional methyl group at C_β. As an example, we identified two peptides T.SAHGNVAEGETKPDPDVTER.C and A.TPLPPT*SAHGNVAEGETKPDPDVTER.C that originate from Hemopexin. The first peptide was successfully cleaved after the CA-modified Thr-29, while the second peptide contains a CA modification at Thr-29 but the cleavage thereof was missed. Even though in the literature only Thr-24 is described to be glycosylated[37], Thr-29 is likely to be also glycosylated because O-glycosylation often occurs on Thr or Ser when a Pro residue is just in front of or three residues behind these Thr or Ser[38]. However, in general, no difference was observed for the cleavage efficiency of CA-modified serines or threonines, neither in respect to missed cleavages nor observed cleavages.

The peptide S.VGAAAGPVVPPCPGR.I (Figure 2.7b) of Fetuin-A, the human orthologue of bovine Fetuin-A which was used for testing before, indicated that the sequence preceding Ser-346 was formerly glycosylated and thus upon the chemical release of the glycan and the CA modification served as a specific cleavage site for Lys-C digestion. Ser-346 was found in the literature to be indeed glycosylated[39].

2.5 Results

The results presented here illustrate the feasibility of the suggested strategy for the enrichment and identification of both N- and O-glycosites.

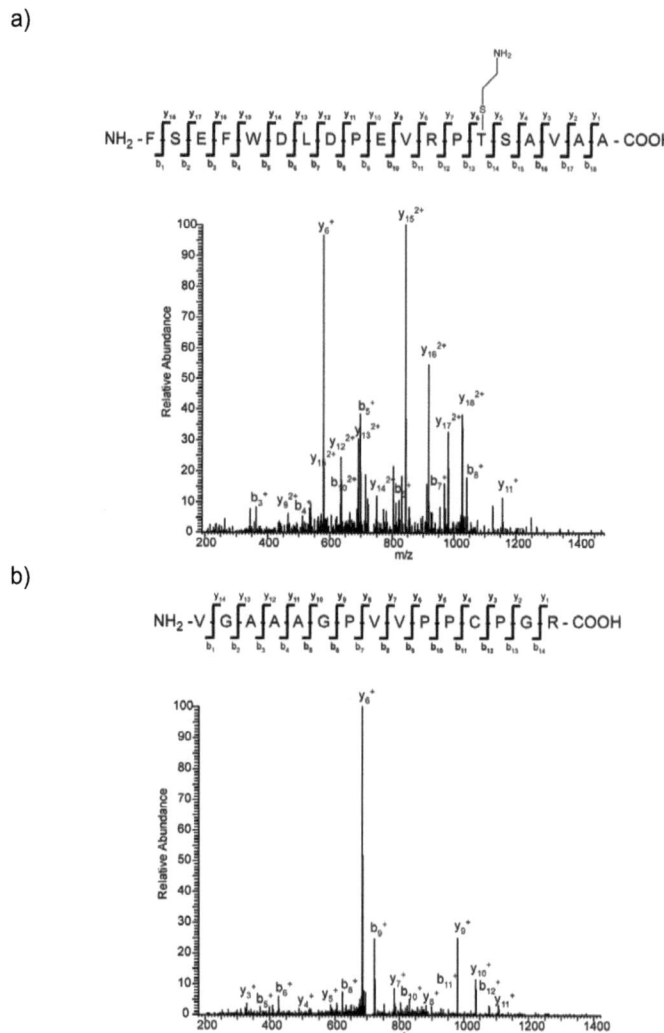

Figure 2.7 MS/MS spectra of two O-glycosites. **a)** CA-modified K.FSEFWDLDPEVRPT*SAVAA.- from Apolipoprotein C-III and **b)** S.VGAAAGPVVPPCPGR.I, a specific cleavage product of an O-glycosite originating from human Alpha-2-HS-glycoprotein (Fetuin-A).

2.6 Discussion

Covalent processing events that change the properties of a protein by proteolytic cleavage or by addition of a modifying group to one or more amino acids are important modulator of protein activity and thus heavily influence cell signaling[40]. While most protein modifications like phosphorylation[41], acetylation[42], N-glycosylation[12], and many others have been extensively studied in the past, large-scale studies on the localization of O-linked glycosylation are lacking. In comparison with N-glycosylation, O-glycosylation is more difficult to study because a consensus sequence around the carbohydrate attachment site has not been identified and for a paucity of enzymes that remove the modification from proteins and peptides. O-linked glycans can be attached to the peptide chain through an O-glycosidic bond to the side chain of serine, threonine, hydroxylysine, or hydroxyproline[43]. O-linked glycosylation is mainly a post-translational event and no precursor is required for protein transfer. Therefore, only exposed amino acid residues will be glycosylated.

We decided to combine the selective enrichment of glycoproteins using hydrazide chemistry and the release of O-glycopeptides via β-elimination. In order to be able to identify the former O-linked glycosylation site, we combined the elimination reaction with a Michael addition of CA, which leads to a mass increment of formerly glycosylated serines and threonines and introduces a trypsin cleavage site. First, chemical conditions were optimized and tested using a synthetic glycopeptide with a single GlcNAc attached to a serine residue. After optimal conditions for the release of the glycan and the modification of its former attachment site were established, the approach was successfully applied to bovine Fetuin-A, a glycoprotein that contains both N- and O-glycosylation sites. All three sites of N-glycosylation and more importantly all five O-glycosylation sites could be unambiguously assigned through either a CA-modified serine or threonine, a specifically generated cleavage site that was proteolysed by Lys-C, or both. Importantly, proteins mixtures containing both O-glycosylation and phosphorylation have to be treated with phosphatases because phosphorylated serines and threonines undergo β-elimination and CA modification alike and thus no conclusion if the site of interest was phosphorylated or glycosylated could be drawn. We have demonstrated with a monophosphopeptide that dephosphorylation can circumvent this problem.

Finally, the method was applied to blood serum samples where N- and O-glycosites were isolated and identified consecutively. The additional tryptic cleavage site generated by CA-modified serines and threonines was computationally challenging. The total number of tryptic termini is an important scoring factor to sort out false positive and true positive database search results[34]. To circumvent the problem, we performed no enzyme constraint database searches and used conservative cutoff values for the scoring parameters returned by the database search engine. Nevertheless, the problem has been well recognized and efforts are already undertaken to solve the issue. When comparing the search results for the N-glycosites using expectation maximization for the calculation of peptide probabilities (PeptideProphet) with the ones obtained by using database search cutoffs, the overall number of peptides identified stayed more or less constant. The lower specificity of 79% using cutoffs compared to the almost 88% achieved by PeptideProphet can be explained by the use of the N-glycosylation motif information by PeptideProphet, which it uses to gain additional confidence.

The final results of the blood serum glycoprotein analysis revealed that a relatively small overlap between N- and O-glycoproteins was achieved. Out of the 50 O-glycoproteins identified in this experiment, four were found to be among the O-glycoproteins and thus both N- and O-glycosylated. When comparing the 50 O-glycoprotein to all the proteins contained in UniPep (5781 entries), a resource of N-glycoproteins, another 9 proteins were found to be N-glycosylated. Interestingly, O-glycosites of 9 different mucins were detected. The heavily O-glycosylated mucins, which carry clusters of GalNAc-based glycans in repetitive Ser- and Thr-rich peptides, have suggested the term 'mucin-type' to designate this complex class of O-linked oligosaccharides[35]. Among the mucins identified was also the Ovarian carcinoma antigen CA125, a biomarker used in blood-based ovarian cancer screening[44]. This and the fact that previously known O-glycosylation sites were identified suggest that our strategy is indeed enriching for the O-glyco-proteome that was targeted.

The strategy for the concurrent identification of N- and O-linked glycoproteins is thought to facilitate further biomarker discovery research. It has been already shown for N-glycoprotein enrichment based tissue and blood serum profiling as well as for cell surface glycoprotein analysis that the reduction in sample complexity greatly alleviates protein discovery and quantification thereof. We believe that analyzing the O-glycoproteins in addition will extend glyco-proteome coverage as well as supporting already identified glycoproteins by contributing additional glycosites and thus strengthen their evidence.

2.7 References

1. Aebersold, R.H. & Goodlett, D.R. Mass spectrometry in proteomics. *Chem Rev* **101**, 269-95 (2001).
2. Brunner, E. et al. A high-quality catalog of the Drosophila melanogaster proteome. *Nat Biotechnol* **25**, 576-83 (2007).
3. Baerenfaller, K. et al. Genome-Scale Proteomics Reveals Arabidopsis thaliana Gene Models and Proteome Dynamics. *Science* (2008).
4. Brand, J., Haslberger, T., Zolg, W., Pestlin, G. & Palme, S. Depletion efficiency and recovery of trace markers from a multiparameter immunodepletion column. *Proteomics* **6**, 3236-42 (2006).
5. Issaq, H.J., Chan, K.C., Janini, G.M., Conrads, T.P. & Veenstra, T.D. Multidimensional separation of peptides for effective proteomic analysis. *J Chromatogr B Analyt Technol Biomed Life Sci* **817**, 35-47 (2005).
6. Gygi, S.P. et al. Quantitative analysis of complex protein mixtures using isotope-coded affinity tags. *Nat Biotechnol* **17**, 994-9 (1999).
7. Bodenmiller, B., Mueller, L.N., Mueller, M., Domon, B. & Aebersold, R.H. Reproducible isolation of distinct, overlapping segments of the phosphoproteome. *Nat Methods* **4**, 231-7 (2007).

2 - Selective isolation and MS-based identification of O-linked glycopeptides

8. Zhang, H., Li, X.J., Martin, D.B. & Aebersold, R.H. Identification and quantification of N-linked glycoproteins using hydrazide chemistry, stable isotope labeling and mass spectrometry. *Nat Biotechnol* 21, 660-6 (2003).
9. Kumar, S. et al. Global analysis of protein tyrosine phosphatase activity with ultra-sensitive fluorescent probes. *J Proteome Res* 5, 1898-905 (2006).
10. Kratchmarova, I., Blagoev, B., Haack-Sorensen, M., Kassem, M. & Mann, M. Mechanism of divergent growth factor effects in mesenchymal stem cell differentiation. *Science* 308, 1472-7 (2005).
11. Gahmberg, C.G. & Tolvanen, M. Why mammalian cell surface proteins are glycoproteins. *Trends Biochem Sci* 21, 308-11 (1996).
12. Zhang, H. et al. High throughput quantitative analysis of serum proteins using glycopeptide capture and liquid chromatography mass spectrometry. *Mol Cell Proteomics* 1, 791-804 (2002).
13. Pan, S. et al. High throughput proteome screening for biomarker detection. *Mol Cell Proteomics* 4, 182-90 (2005).
14. Hägglund, P. et al. An enzymatic deglycosylation scheme enabling identification of core fucosylated N-glycans and O-glycosylation site mapping of human plasma proteins. *J Proteome Res* 6, 3021-31 (2007).
15. Edge, A.S. Deglycosylation of glycoproteins with trifluoromethanesulphonic acid: elucidation of molecular structure and function. *Biochem J* 376, 339-50 (2003).
16. Wells, L. et al. Mapping sites of O-GlcNAc modification using affinity tags for serine and threonine post-translational modifications. *Mol Cell Proteomics* 1, 791-804 (2002).
17. Huang, Y., Konse, T., Mechref, Y. & Novotny, M.V. Matrix-assisted laser desorption/ionization mass spectrometry compatible beta-elimination of O-linked oligosaccharides. *Rapid Commun Mass Spectrom* 16, 1199-204 (2002).
18. Rusnak, F., Zhou, H. & Hathaway, G.M. Identification of phosphorylated and glycosylated sites in peptides by chemically targeted proteolysis. *J Biomol Tech* 13, 228-237 (2002).
19. Pedrioli, P.G. et al. A common open representation of mass spectrometry data and its application to proteomics research. *Nat Biotechnol* 22, 1459-66 (2004).
20. Eng, J.K., McCormack, A.L. & Yates, J.R. An approach to correlate tandem mass spectral data of peptides with amino acid sequences in a protein database. *J Am Soc Mass Spectrom* 5, 976-89 (1994).
21. Keller, A., Eng, J.K., Zhang, N., Li, X.J. & Aebersold, R.H. A uniform proteomics MS/MS analysis platform utilizing open XML file formats. *Mol Syst Biol* 1, 2005.0017 (2005).
22. Oda, Y., Nagasu, T. & Chait, B.T. Enrichment analysis of phosphorylated proteins as a tool for probing the phosphoproteome. *Nat Biotechnol* 19, 379-82 (2001).
23. Meyer, H.E., Hoffmann-Posorske, E., Korte, H. & Heilmeyer, L.M. Sequence analysis of phosphoserine-containing peptides. Modification for picomolar sensitivity. *FEBS Lett* 204, 61-6 (1986).
24. Simpson, D.L., Hranisavljevic, J. & Davidson, E.A. Elimination and sulfite addition as a means of localization and identification of substituted seryl and threonyl residues in proteins and proteoglycans. *Biochemistry* 11, 1849-56 (1972).
25. Adamczyk, M., Gebler, J.C. & Wu, J. Selective analysis of phosphopeptides within a protein mixture by chemical modification, reversible biotinylation and mass spectrometry. *Rapid Commun Mass Spectrom* 15, 1481-8 (2001).
26. Goshe, M.B. et al. Phosphoprotein isotope-coded affinity tag approach for isolating and quantitating phosphopeptides in proteome-wide analyses. *Anal Biochem* 73, 2578-86 (2001).
27. Byford, M.F. Rapid and selective modification of phosphoserine residues catalysed by Ba2+ ions for their detection during peptide microsequencing. *Biochem J* 280 (Pt 1), 261-5 (1991).
28. Knight, Z.A. et al. Phosphospecific proteolysis for mapping sites of protein phosphorylation. *Nat Biotechnol* 21, 1047-54 (2003).
29. Kelly, W.G., Dahmus, M.E. & Hart, G.W. RNA polymerase II is a glycoprotein. Modification of the COOH-terminal domain by O-GlcNAc. *J Biol Chem* 268, 10416-24 (1993).
30. Rademaker, G.J. et al. Mass spectrometric determination of the sites of O-glycan attachment with low picomolar sensitivity. *Anal Biochem* 257, 149-60 (1998).
31. Rusnak, F., Zhou, J. & Hathaway, G.M. Reaction of phosphorylated and O-glycosylated peptides by chemically targeted identification at ambient temperature. *J Biomol Tech* 15, 296-304 (2004).
32. Pisano, A. et al. Identifying sites of glycosylation in proteins. *Techniques in Glycobiology*, 648 (1997).
33. Wilkinson, J.M. & Darbre, A. Fragmentation of polypeptides by enzymic methods (1986).
34. Keller, A., Nesvizhskii, A.I., Kolker, E. & Aebersold, R.H. Empirical statistical model to estimate the accuracy of peptide identifications made by MS/MS and database search. *Anal Chem* 74, 5383-92 (2002).
35. Hanisch, F.G. O-glycosylation of the mucin type. *Biol Chem* 382, 143-9 (2001).
36. Brewer, H.B., Shulman, R., Herbert, P., Ronan, R. & Wehrly, K. The complete amino acid sequence of alanine apolipoprotein (apoC-3), and apolipoprotein from human plasma very low density lipoproteins. *J Biol Chem* 249, 4975-84 (1974).
37. Takahashi, N., Takahashi, Y. & Putnam, F.W. Structure of human hemopexin: O-glycosyl and N-glycosyl sites and unusual clustering of tryptophan residues. *Proc Natl Acad Sci USA* 81, 2021-5 (1984).
38. Van den Steen, P.E., Rudd, P.M., Dwek, R.A. & Opdenakker, G. Concepts and principles of O-linked glycosylation. *Crit Rev Biochem Mol Biol* 33, 151-208 (1998).

2.7 References

39. Gejyo, F. et al. Characterization of the B-chain of human plasma alpha 2HS-glycoprotein. The complete amino acid sequence and primary structure of its heteroglycan. *J Biol Chem* **258**, 4966-71 (1983).
40. Mann, M. & Jensen, O.N. Proteomic analysis of post-translational modifications. *Nat Biotechnol* **21**, 255-61 (2003).
41. Bodenmiller, B. et al. PhosphoPep--a phosphoproteome resource for systems biology research in Drosophila Kc167 cells. *Mol Syst Biol* **3**, 139 (2007).
42. Beck, H.C. et al. Quantitative proteomic analysis of post-translational modifications of human histones. *Mol Cell Proteomics* **5**, 1314-25 (2006).
43. Dwek, R.A., Edge, C.J., Harvey, D.J., Wormald, M.R. & Parekh, R.B. Analysis of glycoprotein-associated oligosaccharides. *Annu Rev Biochem* **62**, 65-100 (1993).
44. Jacobs, I.J. & Menon, U. Progress and challenges in screening for early detection of ovarian cancer. *Mol Cell Proteomics* **3**, 355-66 (2004).

3 Phenotyping cells without antibodies: MS identification and quantitation of N-linked cell surface glycoproteins

3.1 Authorship

This chapter describes shared work with Bernd Wollscheid, Damaris Bausch-Fluck, Christine Henderson, Robert O'Brien, Ruedi Aebersold, Julian D. Watts. The work presented here describes the methodology to enrich for cell surface glycoproteins and lays the basis for the next chapter where I applied the technique in a quantitative approach to detect specific changes in the cell surface glyco-proteome. My contribution to this work was to proof that the enrichment is not biased to high sialic acid content glycans and that the method works reproducibly. This chapter represents an adaptation of the following research article: Wollscheid, B et al., *Nature Biotechnology* **27**, 378-86 (2009)[1].

3.2 Summary

The classification of cell types has relied on the identification of cell surface proteins as differentiation markers. Currently, flow cytometry allows for the detection of up to a dozen differentiation markers in a single measurement. We have developed a methodology for the multiplexed, quantitative, mass-spectrometric identification of cell surface glycoproteins, and their N-glycosites, which can be used to phenotype cells without antibodies, in an unbiased fashion, and without *a priori* knowledge. The cell surface capturing (CSC) technology allows for the isolation, identification and quantification of N-glycosites from the extracellular domains of cell surface proteins in a discovery-driven mode. Several hundred *bona fide* cell surface glycoproteins and their N-glycosites, including CD-annotated and novel proteins, can be identified in a single MS experiment. CSC technology enables a more comprehensive view of the cell surface glycoprotein landscape, and can detect glycoproteins as potential differentiation markers that are currently not accessible by other means.

3.3 Introduction

The molecular composition of the plasma membrane (PM) and its dynamic changes, determine how a cell can interact with its environment at any given moment. Proteins embedded in the membrane that have exposed, extracellular domains are crucial for cell-cell communication, interaction with pathogens, binding of chemical messengers, and responses to environmental perturbations[2, 3]. Due to the fact that cell surface proteins confer specific cellular functions, and that they are easily accessible, they are often used as markers for the classification of cell types[4] and as drug targets[5]. By using available antibodies against cell surface proteins, cells are thus often classified or immunophenotyped according to their cell surface protein expression profile[6]. This approach has successfully been used by immunologists for the immunophenotyping cells of the immune system, and for the development of the cluster of differentiation (CD) nomenclature for antibodies against cell surface molecules, which has been used as the classification basis of the ~220 currently known cell types[7]. Despite these successes, most cell surface proteins remain undetectable due to a lack of suitable antibodies[8]. A comparison of the relatively small number of available CD cell surface protein markers (~320), with the number of predicted human transmembrane proteins (~13'000), or the 3'094 membrane glycoproteins currently annotated in UniProt, illustrates the gap between the available and potential cell surface markers[9, 10]. Furthermore, due to a lack of enabling technology, cell surface protein analysis has been limited to the measurement of about 12 CD molecules in parallel. Finally, the development of a new CD assay is time consuming and expensive since, in each case, an optimal antibody needs to be selected, and cell surface expression for the target protein needs to be tested and validated by flow cytometry or immunohistochemistry[11]. Therefore, in spite of its successes, the current gold-standard approach for cell classification via CD profiling has substantial limitations.

Currently, it is not known how many different proteins are expressed on the surface of a particular cell, and at what levels they are expressed[12]. In cases in which copy numbers of proteins are published, these values are often not measured from the same cell type, and are imprecise due to variations in antibody affinities. Similarly, inferring quantitative cell surface protein data from gene transcript measurements is also problematic. Transcript microarrays can accurately predict neither the quantity, nor the specific cellular location of the corresponding proteins[12]. Quantitative PCR of selected mRNAs from suspected or *bona fide* cell surface expressed proteins can reveal up- or down-regulation of specific transcripts, but does not support statements about their translation, or cellular location of the final product. Thus in order to more fully and reliably characterize cell types via their cell surface proteome, new experimental approaches are required.

3 - Cell surface capturing of N-linked glycoproteins 47

Mass-spectrometry (MS) based proteomics allows for the sensitive, parallel identification and quantification of significant numbers of peptides/proteins[13, 14]. To date, the identification of the cell surface proteome by quantitative MS has been hampered by the difficulty of obtaining homogenous and highly enriched plasma membrane protein isolates, the limited relative abundance of surface membrane proteins, compared with cytoskeletal or cytosolic components, and the difficulty in resolving and identifying hydrophobic proteins and peptides[15, 16]. Commonly, analyses of the cell surface proteome are attempted by first enriching plasma membrane proteins by subcellular fractionation, with subsequent mass spectrometric analysis of these isolates[17-19]. Such studies typically identify a small percentage of *bona fide* cell surface proteins that are largely contaminated with other proteins, specifically those from intracellular membranes. The direct experimental identification of membrane surface proteins by mass spectrometry therefore remains a considerable challenge.

In an attempt to overcome the specificity problem for membrane surface protein analysis, chemical tagging strategies have been used in conjunction with subcellular fractionation. Specifically, biotinylation of lysine residues of the extracellular domains of plasma membrane proteins has been a popular choice to identify cell surface proteins[20-22]. Other approaches have included selected known peptide monitoring[23], lectin-based methods[24, 25], cell surface shaving[26], two phase separation[27], and antibody-mediated membrane enrichment[28] strategies. Although all of these methods are able to identify membrane proteins to some extent, they still lack the specificity and selectivity needed for conclusive and comprehensive analysis of the surface membrane proteome.

In 2003, we developed a novel approach for the selective isolation of N-glycosites (sites of N-glycosylation in their de-glycosylated form)[29] from glycoproteins in blood serum and from cellular samples. The method proved to be very specific, and led to an increased sensitivity in glycoprotein identifications in complex samples, due to the reduction of sample complexity. Since most cell surface proteins and secreted proteins are known or predicted to be glycosylated, we sought to adapt this technology to selective identification of cell surface glycoproteins[30]. The cell surface capturing (CSC) technology that we have thus developed and present here now makes possible, for the first time, the comprehensive and quantitative analysis of the cell surface glycoprotein landscape at very high specificity. This technology will be useful for the identification of new cell surface protein targets for drug development, for the improved classification of cell types, and generally, for better understanding of the cell surface proteome and its function.

3.4 Experimental Procedures

Harvesting of cells and oxidation of cell surface glycoproteins. 5×10^7 cells (Jurkat T, Ramos B or Drosophila Kc167 cells) were collected in a 50 ml tube and washed two times with labeling buffer (PBS pH 6.5, 0.1% FBS). Subsequently, cells were oxidized for 10 min in the dark at 4°C with 1.6 mM sodium-meta-periodate (#20504, Piercenet.com). The cell pellet was washed two times with 50 ml labeling buffer to remove residual sodium-meta-periodate and to deplete dead cells/fragments. In control experiments, cells were treated with 100 mU of Neuraminidase (Sigma, N2876) in PBS at 37°C for 30 min to remove terminal sialic acid residues before CSC labeling.

Cell surface labeling. The cell pellet was resuspended in 10 ml labeling buffer containing 5 mM biocytin hydrazide (#90060, Biotium.com) for 60 min at 4°C on a rotator on slow speed. Upon labeling, the cell pellet was washed two times with 50 ml labeling buffer to remove unreacted biocytin hydrazide and to deplete dead cells/fragments.

Cell lysis and membrane preparation. The cell pellet was resuspended in 12 ml detergent free, ice-cold, hypotonic lysis buffer (10 mM Tris pH 7.5, 0.5 M $MgCl_2$). After 10 min on ice, cells were homogenized with forty strokes using a Dounce homogenizer (Wheaton, USA, 15 ml Dounce Tissue Grinder). Upon homogenization, an equal volume of membrane prep buffer (280 mM sucrose, 50 mM MES pH 6.0, 450 mM NaCl, 10 mM $MgCl_2$) was added to the lysate. After 10 min the lysate was centrifuged at 2500xg at 4°C for 10 min. The homogenization procedure was repeated one more time with the pellet. The combined supernatants (the membrane fraction) was centrifuged in an Ultracentrifuge (Beckmann Ultacentrifuge L8-M Ultra; Beckmann SW41 swing rotor, 6x12 ml tubes; #344059; Beckmann Ultra Clear Centrifuge tubes; 12 ml) at 35'000rpm for one hour at 4°C. Upon centrifugation the pellet was incubated with 0.025M Na_2CO_3, (pH 11) for thirty min on ice and the ultracentrifugation step was repeated once.

Digestion of labeled membrane preparation. The pellet was resuspended in 500 µl 50 mM ammonium bicarbonate (Sigma) containing 0.05% of the acid-labile surfactant RapiGest (#186001860,Waters.com). The membrane preparation was indirectly sonicated in continous mode at 100% for 10min in a VialTweeter (hielscher.com) in order to obtain a translucent solution. The proteins were digested for four hours with LysC (#324715, Calbiochem) and subsequently overnight with trypsin (#V5113, Promega). Upon digestion, the peptide mixture was boiled for 10 min to inactivate the proteases and protease inhibitors were added (#11873580001, Roche Complete tabs).

Glycopeptide capture. 1 ml of UltraLink Streptavidin Plus beads (#53117, Piercenet.com) were washed twice with 50 mM ammonium bicarbonate in Mobicols (#M3009, Bocascientific.com). The

3 - Cell surface capturing of N-linked glycoproteins 49

peptide mixture was added to the beads and incubated for one hour in a MacsMix head over head shaker (#130-090-753, Miltenyi Biotec). The captured glycopeptides were washed intensively with 0.5 Triton X-100 (Sigma) in 50mM Ammoniumbicarbonate; followed by 10 ml 5 M sodium chloride, followed by 10 ml 100 mM sodium carbonate pH 11.0, followed by 10 ml 100 mM Ammonium bicarbonate. Washing was performed in Mobicols connected to a Vac-ManLaboratory Vacuum Manifold (Promega).

Release of N-linked glycopeptides. Washed beads were incubated in 600 µl Ammonium-bicarbonate containing PNGase F (NEB) overnight in a head-over-head shaker at 37°C. Upon incubation, the beads were washed once with 500 µl 50 mM Ammoniumbicarbonat and once with 20% Acetonitrile. Eluates were combined and dried in a speedvac for subsequent LC-MS/MS analysis. In control experiments, PNGase A (SIGMA, G0535) was used according to the manufactures instructions.

LC-MS and database analysis. Peptides were re-solubilized in 0.1% formic acid and analyzed via nanospray liquid chromatography tandem mass spectrometry (LC-MS/MS). LCQ DECA XP ion trap, LTQ and LTQ-FT mass spectrometers (Thermoelectron, San Jose, CA) were used with HP 1100/1200 solvent delivery systems (Agilent, Polo Alto, CA). Peptides were pressure-loaded or loaded via an autosampler on a capillary reverse-phase C18 column (75 µm i.d. and 12 cm of bed length; 200 Å, 5-µm C18 beads, Michrom BioResources Inc). Peptides were eluted from the capillary column at a flow rate of 180 nl/min to the mass spectrometer through an integrated nanospray emitter tip. Needle voltage was set to 2.0 kV. The mobile phase used for a linear gradient elution of 15-35% B in 45 min followed by 35-70% B in 15 min consisted of (A) 0.1% formic acid (B) 100% acetonitrile. Both MS and MS/MS spectra were acquired with the instrument operating in the data-dependent mode of one MS scan followed by three MS/MS scans. Ion signals above a predetermined threshold automatically triggered the instrument to switch from MS to MS/MS mode for generating collision-induced dissociation (CID) spectra. All MS/MS spectra were searched against the International Protein Index (IPI) database (Version 3.26) using the SEQUEST algorithm. Statistical analysis of the data was performed by using a combination of ISB open source software tools (PeptideProphet, ProteinProphet). A ProteinProphet protein probability score ≥ 0.9 was used to filter the data, followed by manual validation. Quantitative data analysis was performed using the XPRESS software[19]. Data was imported, stored, annotated and validated within the SISYPHUS database software. Identified proteins within the CSC dataset were validated and "contaminations" were singled out in a bioinformatic process, yielding 100% *bona fide* cell surface labeled glycoproteins. This bioinformatic process was developed and validates the CSC protein identifications by using four criteria. [1] A ProteinProphet Protein Probability cutoff is set depending on the individual data quality of the dataset, limiting the false positive protein identification rate to below 1% [2] All identified proteins were analyzed with two transmembrane prediction algorithms (SOSUI, TMHMM) indicating hydrophobic protein sequence regions. CSC proteins must have one or more transmembrane segments (exception: GPI linkage). [3] All proteins must be identified with at least one peptide containing the consensus NxS/T glycosylation motif. [4] Every identified glycopeptide must have an asparagine to aspartic acid deamidation site with a MS measured mass difference of 0.986 Da, indicating the cell surface labeling and the enzymatic deamidation during the CSC workflow. If all four criteria match we can be confident that the CSC MS identified protein was at the cell surface at the time of the CSC labeling. Please note that this statement can be made solely on the basis of the generated data in combination with bioinformatic tools without consulting public protein databases and their annotations.

FACS. Flow cytometric analysis was performed on CSC labeled lymphocytes. Cells labeled with biocytin hydrazide were incubated with Streptavidin Alexa Fluor 488 (#S-11223, Molecular Probes) at 4°C for 20 min. Labeled cells were washed twice and analyzed using a FACScan (BD Biosciences) in combination with CellQuest software.

CONFOCAL IMAGING. In order to detect labeled cell surface glycoproteins, cells were stained for 20 min with Streptavidin Alexa Fluor 488 at 1:100 dilution in blocking solution and washed with PBS. Upon washing, cells were transfered onto coverslides and fixed with 4% paraformaldehyde for 10 min and subsequently washed with PBS. The nucleus was counterstained for five min with 1 µg/ml DAPI (Merck) and washed with PBS. In order to detect labeled cell surface glycoproteins and potentially labeled intracellular glycoproteins, cells were permeabilized for 5 min with 0.1% saponin. Permeabilized cells were stained for 20 min with Streptavidin Alexa Fluor 488 at 1:100 dilution in blocking solution and washed with PBS. In control experiments, Neuraminidase treated and untreated cells were stained with peanut agglutinin-Rhodamine (Axxora, VC-RL-1072) according to the manufacturers instructions. Coverslides were mounted with Fluoromount-G (Southern Biotechnology). Confocal laser scan microscopy images were taken with a 64x1.4 oil objective using a Leica TCS SP2 AOBS and filters as follows: AF488 emission 501-554 nm, excitation 490 nm, DAPI emission 409-478 nm, excitation 365 nm. Images were merged with Photoshop 6.0 and LCS Lite (Leica) software.

CELL CULTURE. Human Ramos B cells and Jurkat T cells were cultivated in RPMI1640 supplemented with 10% FCS, 100 Units of Pen/Strep and 0.1 mM ß-mercaptoethanol (Invitrogen.com). SILAC labeling of cells was performed according to the manufacturer's instruction (Invitrogen.com). CD3/CD28 co-stimulation was performed as previously described[31].

3 - Cell surface capturing of N-linked glycoproteins

3.5 Results

3.5.1 Strategy for the selective identification of cell surface exposed N-glycosites

The goal of this project was to develop a technology for selective mass-spectrometric identification of cell surface glycoproteins and their quantification, i.e. for cell surface scanning. We thus designed and applied a strategy of selective chemical tagging of cell surface glycoproteins on the intact, living cell, followed by high-affinity enrichment and gel-free LC-MS/MS analysis of peptides derived from the tagged proteins (Figure 3.1). In more detail, the overall CSC approach utilizes a multi-step, tandem affinity labeling strategy to confer the desired specificity for cell surface glycoproteins. The specific steps of the procedure are: i) gentle, covalent chemical labeling of oxidized carbohydrate-containing proteins on live cells using the bi-functional linker molecule, biocytin hydrazide (BH)[32, 33]; ii) affinity enrichment of BH labeled peptides; iii) specific enzymatic peptide release that allows for systematic and selective identification of N-glycosites from the surface glycoproteins; iv) subsequent peptide and protein identification via reversed phase capillary liquid chromatography, coupled to tandem mass spectrometry (LC-MS/MS).

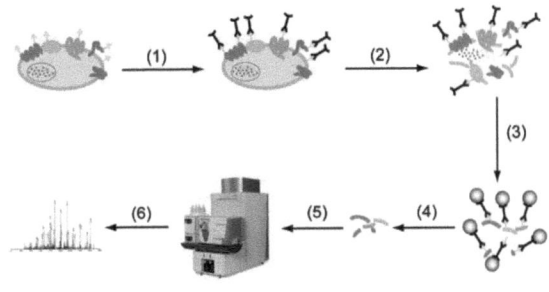

Figure 3.1 The cell-surface capturing technology (CSC) utilizes a multi-step tandem affinity labeling strategy to confer the desired specificity for the glycoproteins on the cell surface. These steps are (1) Tagging of reactive groups from PM proteins (yellow triangles: glycans; black: bi-functional linker molecules); (2) Cell homogenization; (3) Protein digestion and affinity purification; (4) Peptide release; (5) Peptide analysis by LC-MS/MS; (6) Peptide/ protein identification.

The key difference to other published approaches, and which leads to the superior selectivity of the present method for cell surface proteins, is the oxidation of cell surface polysaccharides on living cells, in combination with subsequent BH labeling. CSC technology is geared towards the identification of glycoproteins through the detection of tryptic N-glycosite containing peptides (> 9 AA) from extracellular domains of glycoproteins. The reaction conditions were carefully optimized in dose response and time curve experiments to both maximize for cell viability, as judged by the integrity of the cells in the forward/sideward scatter in combination with Propidiumiodide uptake, and to prevent side reactions from the uncatalyzed oxidation agent. Harsher oxidation conditions to label specifically cell surface glycoproteins using higher concentrations of Sodium periodate (> 2.5 mM) led to increased cell death (depending on the celltype) and therefore labeling could not be restricted to the cell surface, as judged by FACS, IHC and MS analysis (data not shown).

3.5.2 The CSC labeling reaction is efficient and selective for glycoproteins

We first examined the labeling efficiency of the CSC technology using the Jurkat human T lymphocyte cell line as a substrate. Cells were oxidized, BH-treated, and subsequently labeled with streptavidin-AF488 to visualize the degree of biotinylation and the localization of the biotin groups added. Results (Figure 3.2, FACS) show homogenous fluorescent labeling. In contrast, only a slight increase in fluorescence intensity could be observed after BH treatment in the absence of oxidation of the cells (colored yellow), indicating very few cell surface BH-available aldehyde- or keto-groups prior to oxidation treatment, compared with the untreated cells (colored red). The CSC labeling conditions were optimized for efficient labeling, while maintaining maximum viability of the cells.

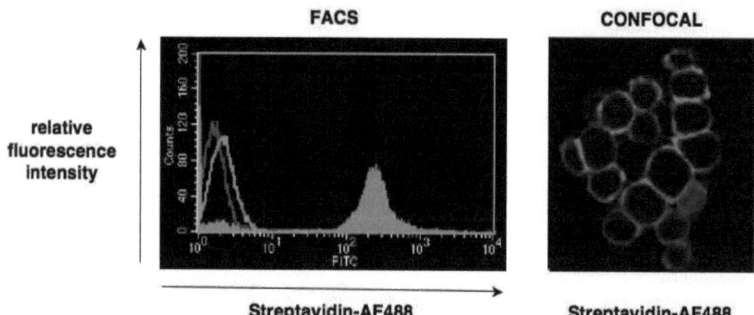

Figure 3.2 The CSC reaction is selective for glycans on the cell surface. FACS: Three Jurkat T lymphocyte populations are shown in this ungated FACS histogram: [RED] control cells; [ORANGE] only biocytin hydrazide; [GREEN] Sodium periodate and biocytin hydrazide treated cells. Streptavidin-AF488 fluorophore was used for detection. CONFOCAL MICROSCOPY: Confocal images of Jurkat T lymphocytes upon visualization of the tagged cell surface polysaccarides. Cells were oxidized, BH labeled and upon permeabilisation incubated with Streptavidin-AF488 [Green].

3 - Cell surface capturing of N-linked glycoproteins

We next investigated the specificity of the cell surface labeling. Jurkat cells were again oxidized and labeled with BH, then additionally permeabilized prior to streptavidin-AF488 treatment. Cells were then visualized using a confocal microscope (Figure 3.2, Confocal). The distribution of the streptavidin fluorescent dye in the central cellular stack section of labeled cells confirmed that the CSC labeling was specific for the cell surface, and that the BH reagent was not able to penetrate the cell membranes. We thus concluded that the cell surface of a live cell population could be labeled selectively and homogenously using the CSC approach.

3.5.3 CSC technology enables the selective MS identification of cell surface glycoproteins

We next performed a proof-of-principle CSC experiment where we labeled Jurkat cells as described above, and analyzed the recovered N-glycosites by LC-MS/MS. The measured MS/MS spectra were searched against a human protein sequence database using SEQUEST[34], and the search results were validated using the TransProteomicPipeline (TPP)[35]. The results were then imported into a cell surface protein atlas. In this way, 110 proteins were identified from ~5×10^7 Jurkat T lymphocytes, at a ProteinProphet protein probability[36] of ≥ 0.9 (see Supplementary Table S3.1), which, for this dataset, represented a false discovery rate of < 1%. Of these, 104 proteins (95%) were CSC labeled cell surface glycoproteins, and included 43 CD annotated proteins, providing a broad view of the specific Jurkat T lymphocyte surface glycoprotein landscape and the corresponding N-glycosites (visualized in Figure 3.3 via CYTOSCAPE[37]). Jurkat T lymphocytes treated with Neuramidase to eliminate terminal sialic acid residues yielded a similar number of glycoprotein identifications by using the CSC technology (data not shown). Furthermore, a control PNGase A treatment of bead-bound glycopeptides from human Jurkat T cells led to no N-glycosite identifications, indicating that PNGase A cleavable 3-linked fucose structures do not exist on Jurkat T cells or are rare and potential N-glycosites are below the MS detection limit. The CSC technology was further applied to Drosophila cells (Kc167) were no sialic acid can be detected[38]. 91 cell surface glycoproteins were identified through 210 N-glycosites (92% specificity for N-glycosites) indicating that the CSC technology is not dependent on sialic acid residues.

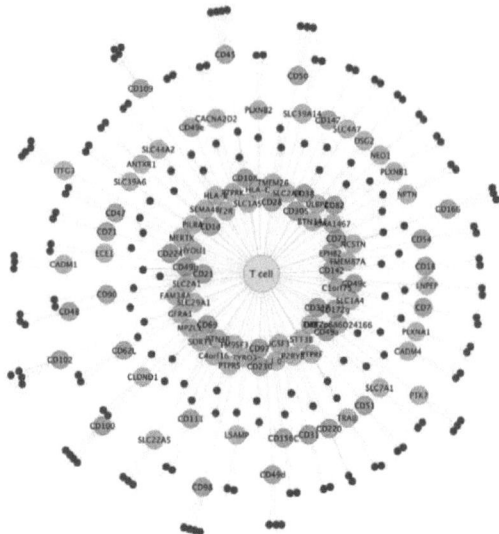

Figure 3.3 Jurkat T lymphocyte surface glyco-proteome. CSC identified glycoproteins and their glycosites from Jurkat T lymphocytes [yellow middle circle: Jurkat cell; red circles: CD proteins (label:CD number); green circles: non CD annotated proteins (label: ENTREZ gene id); blue circles: glycopeptides containg glycosylation motif]. Glycoproteins towards the outside of the spring embedded Cytoscape view have more unique CSC identified glycopeptides containing an NxS/T motif.

The CSC strategy proved to be very robust, and significantly more selective for MS-based identification of cell surface glycoproteins than previously published methods. The 104 CSC identified proteins in Jurkat T cells covered a wide range of PANTHER[39] molecular functions, pathways, and biological processes, indicating that the CSC technology could, in a single analysis, perform a more comprehensive view of the cell surface proteome than previously possible in multiple experiments (Figure 3.4, see Supplementary Table S3.1). In this dataset, for example, high abundance proteins such as CD98, as well as low abundance receptors such as the G-protein coupled receptor P2Y purinoceptor 8, were confidently identified. Also, among the CSC identified proteins, were receptor phosphatases such as CD45, and receptor tyrosine kinases such as TYRO3. The CSC technology also identified single transmembrane as well as multi-transmembrane containing proteins. Indeed, cell surface transmembrane domain-containing glycoproteins identified from the Jurkat T lymphocytes contained a range from one to twenty-five TMHMM[40] predicted transmembrane domains (see Supplementary Table S3.1). We also noted that many of the proteins in Supplementary Table S3.1 would not be readily detectable by immunology-based methods, due to a lack of specific antibodies.

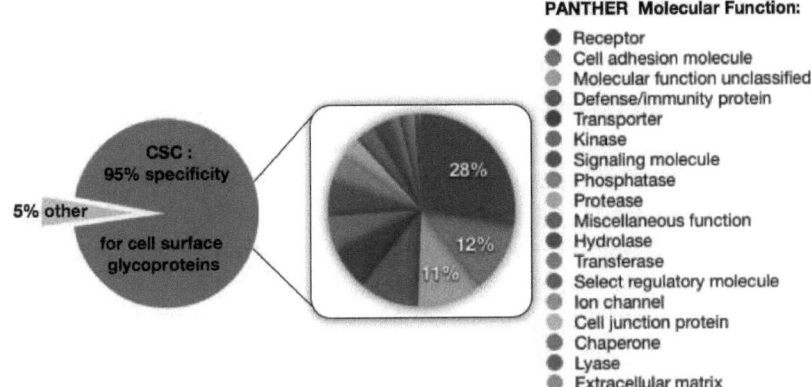

Figure 3.4 Specificity of the CSC technology and molecular function of identified proteins. 110 proteins were identified in a CSC Experiment including 43 CD proteins from Jurkat T lymphocytes with a specificity of 95% for cell surface glycoproteins. 5% were identified non-specifically. The PANTHER molecular function analysis of the 104 cell surface glycoproteins is displayed on the right (see also Supplementary Table 3.1).

These results showed an unprecedented degree of specificity for the detection of cell surface proteins, with <5% of identified proteins resulting from co-isolating intracellular and non-glycosylated proteins. Indeed, five of the six contaminating proteins were identified by only a single unique peptide (see Supplementary Table S3.1), and thus represent lower confidence and potential false-positive identifications. Since a repository for Jurkat T lymphocyte cell surface (or any other cell type) expressed glycoproteins does not exist, and all available antibodies against cell surface proteins have never been tested on these particular cells, many of the proteins identified in this single CSC experiment represent new cell surface glycoprotein identifications for this particular cell type. Finally, since these identified glycoproteins effectively represent a 'snapshot', analogous to a cell surface 'barcode' of the Jurkat cell surface proteome under normal growth conditions, these results also highlighted the potential of the CSC technology for selective and multiplexed MS analysis of cell surface proteins in changing growth, stimulation or disease states, and the quantitative comparison of the resulting patterns.

3.5.4 CSC technology reveals cell surface protein N-glycosite sites and transmembrane protein orientation

The CSC technology is not restricted to the identification of cell surface proteins, it also identifies the specific cell surface protein glycosylation sites. The 110 proteins identified in the experiment described above were inferred from 313 identified peptides. Of these, 289 (92%) were N-glycosites containing the consensus N-glycosylation NxS/T motif (where X is any amino acid, except proline). N-glycosites also showed a predictable fixed mass shift (of 0.984 Da) in the MS and MS/MS spectra as a result of the conversion of glycosylated asparagine to aspartic acid, via the enzymatic deglycosylation step. This mass shift can be observed and confirmed in a mass spectrometer with sufficient mass accuracy, and in so doing, positively identify the N-glycosylation site(s) in the original protein. An example of this is shown in Figure 5 for an N-glycosite from the Anthrax toxin receptor. Since the identified glycosylation site is expected to be on the outside of the PM, the identification of N-glycosites can facilitate the prediction and confirmation of the transmembrane topology of cell surface proteins (data not shown). Data obtained from all our CSC experiments combined have shown that 93.7% of identified glycopeptides contain one NxS/T motif, 6.0% two motifs, and 0.3% have three. We have not identified peptides with four or more glycosylation sites. 60% of identified glycosites are at an NxT motif, with the remaining 40% an NxS motif. Identified cell surface glycosites have a median length of 12 amino acids (AA), and range from 5 to 40 amino acids in length. In turn, the glycoproteins identified via CSC show a range of one to eight unique identified N-glycosites. From these data, we conclude that CSC identified peptides carrying the mass shift signature within the N-glycosylation motif, represent experimentally confirmed cell surface protein N-glycosylation sites.

3 - Cell surface capturing of N-linked glycoproteins 57

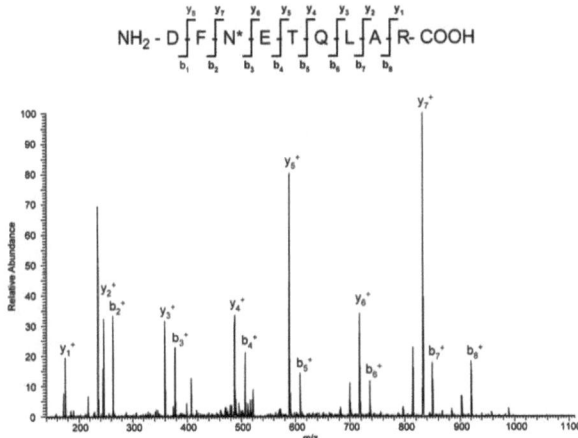

Figure 3.5 Specific MS-based identification of cell surface glycoprotein N-glycosylation sites. Shown is the N-glycosite identification of the CSC peptide DFNETQLAR derived from the Anthrax toxin receptor detected on Jurkat T lymphocytes.

3.5.5 CSC technology is applicable to primary cells, tissues and organs

Since the initial evaluation of the CSC technology was with cultured cell lines, we next set out to assess the performance of the CSC technology on primary cells and tissues. A pre-requisite for the CSC method is that the critical oxidation and cell surface labeling must be done with live cells in solution. Thus successful application to tissues and primary cells would first require getting viable cells into solution. As a proof-of-principle experiment towards this goal, we applied the CSC technology to the identification of cell surface proteins from mouse splenic cells, since protocols for making single cell suspensions of splenocytes from splenic tissues are well established. Upon applying the CSC method to tissue-derived primary mouse splenocytes, we identified 87 proteins at a ProteinProphet protein probability ≥ 0.9 (see Supplementary Table S3.2) and at a false discovery rate of <1%. Of these, 82 proteins (94%) were CSC labeled cell surface proteins, including 38 CD annotated proteins. These 87 proteins were identified via 282 peptides, of which 248 (88%) contained at least one NxS/T motif. As expected, we observed cell surface proteins that were annotated as cell type specific, including known T lymphocyte (e.g. CD3δ and CD8α) and B lymphocyte (e.g. CD22 and CD72) markers, indicating that multiple cell types were present in the primary splenocyte population. Most of the identified cell surface glycoproteins, however, could not be attributed to a specific cell type. In summary, the data showed that the CSC technology is equally applicable to cultured and primary cells, as well as tissues in cases where live single cell suspensions can be generated, such as liver or brain.

3.5.6 CSC technology for quantitative cell surface protein scanning

We next investigated the integration of the CSC technology with quantitative proteomic workflows to detect differences in the cell surface glyco-proteome between related cell types, and upon perturbation of a specific cell type. In the first set of experiments, cultured Ramos B and human Jurkat T human lymphocytes were labeled with isotopically light and heavy SILAC reagents, respectively, and the cell surface glycoproteins were analyzed as previously described. 96 proteins were identified at a ProteinProphet protein probability of ≥ 0.9 and quantified (Supplementary Table S3.3). Of these, 93 (97%) were CSC labeled cell surface glycoproteins, including 40 CD annotated proteins. The 96 proteins were identified via 281 peptides, with 274 peptides (97%) containing one or more NxS/T motif. Quantitative analysis of the signal intensities of the respective isotopically labeled heavy and light peptides also indicated which glycoproteins were expressed on the surface of both cell types in similar amounts (labeled green), which proteins were over-represented on Ramos B, compared with Jurkat T lymphocytes (labeled red), and which proteins were over-represented on the T, compared with B lymphocytes (labeled blue) (Figure 3.6). Selected CSC protein identifications are also indicated in Figure 6 to illustrate the capacity of the quantitative CSC technology to detect relative cell surface protein expression differences for known (and unknown) B and T cell markers. For example CD79b is a component of the B cell receptor which is expressed in B cells but not in T cells[41]. Similarly, CD69 is a well known T cell activation marker[42]. Apart from these known markers, a number of other CD and non-CD annotated glycoproteins showed differential cell surface expression, indicating the different functional capacities of these two cell types (see Supplementary Table S3.3). FACS experiments with a panel of selected antibodies confirmed the CSC detected regulation of glycoproteins on the single cell level (data not shown). The phenotype, and therefore the identity of the B and T cell type under investigation can be deduced from the generated CSC data without using antibodies, and at a far greater level of complexity than is possible with antibodies, in a single experiment. The data thus show that quantitative CSC technology has the capacity to classify cell types at a much higher level of detail, in terms of both the number of markers and the range of marker proteins, than is possible by the conventional use of antibodies.

3 - Cell surface capturing of N-linked glycoproteins 59

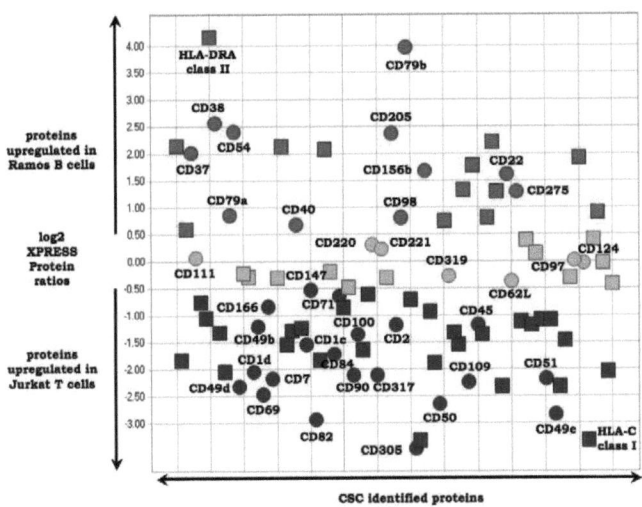

Figure 3.6 Quantitative CSC experiments reveal cell surface glycoproteins differentially expressed on Jurkat T versus Ramos B lymphocytes. Displayed are the XPRESS calculated protein quantitation ratios versus the CSC identified proteins in a SPOTFIRE scatter plot view. Proteins which are present on the cell surface of both cell types in similar amounts are depicted in green. Cell surface proteins which are up-regulated on T cells versus B cells are depicted in blue. Cell surface proteins which are down-regulated in B cells versus T cells are depicted in red. Round shapes indicate proteins which are CD annotated. Square shapes are non CD annotated proteins. Selected CSC identified proteins are labeled. For a list of identified and quantified proteins please see Supplementary Table S3.3.

In a second set of quantitative CSC SILAC experiments, we investigated alterations in the T cell surface glyco-proteome induced by T cell activation[31]. Jurkat T lymphocytes were subjected to co-stimulation with anti-CD3 and anti-CD28 antibodies for 24 hours. 24 hours was chosen based on control FACS experiments showing that the expected up-regulation of the T cell activation marker CD69 was clearly evident at this time point (data not shown). In this experiment 119 proteins were identified and quantified at a ProteinProphet protein probability cutoff of ≥ 0.9 (Supplementary Table S3.4). Of these, 112 proteins (94%) were CSC labeled cell surface proteins, including 47 CD annotated proteins. The 119 proteins were identified via 1,035 peptide identifications, with 920 peptides (88%) containing the NxS/T motif. These results showed, for example, that the CSC SILAC experiment confirmed the strong up-regulation of CD69, and down-regulation of T cell receptor (TCR) cell surface expression upon CD3/CD28 co-stimulation, as would be expected (Figure 3.7)[31]. The data also showed additional up- and down-regulation of a variety of cell surface glycoproteins, some expected, some not previously known, in response to this mode of stimulation, all in a single experiment (data not shown). Indeed, the relative expression changes of 47 different CD proteins were measured at the same time in this MS experiment. In order to assess the accuracy and reproducibility of quantifying cell surface proteome changes detectable by the CSC technology, Schiess et.al.[43] concluded from CSC experiments with *Drosophila* cells that 76% of the quantified features showed a CV equal to or below 30% and the average coefficient of variance of all 1210 aligned features was 24%. For technical replicates CVs between 10% and 13% were achieved. Together, these data demonstrated that quantitative CSC technology allows for the profiling of changes in cell surface marker proteins, upon perturbation of the cellular system, at a much more detailed level than previously possible by conventional methods for cellular phenotyping.

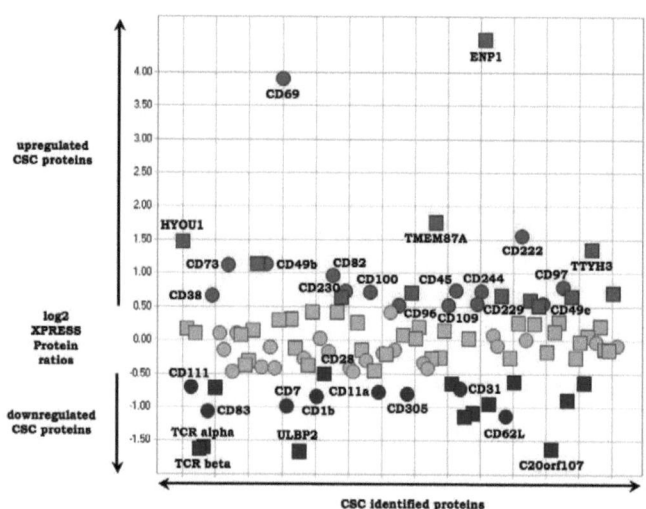

Figure 3.7 Quantitative CSC technology reveals the specific up-regulation and down-regulation of Jurkat T cell proteins upon CD3/CD28 co-stimulation after 24 h. Glycoproteins which are present on the cell surface before and after stimulation in similar amounts are depicted in green. Cell surface glycoproteins which are up-regulated upon T cell stimulation are depicted in red. Cell surface glycoproteins which are down-regulated upon T cell stimulation are depicted in blue. Round shapes indicate proteins which are CD annotated. Square shapes are non CD annotated proteins. Selected CSC identified proteins are labeled. For a list of identified and quantified glycoproteins please see Supplementary Table S3.4 for the respective glycopeptides.

3.6 Discussion

For most cell types, it is not known which proteins are expressed at the cell surface, and how these protein expression patterns are changing quantitatively upon perturbation or differentiation. The paucity of this biologically highly relevant information is for the most part a consequence of a lack of specific antibodies that support the detection of cell surface proteins by immunodetection methods. Such methods, including flow cytometry and immunohistochemistry, have been the mainstay of cell surface protein analysis to date. The generation of antibodies with validated specificity remains a major hurdle for such studies, and the establishment of multiplexed assays for identification of sets of cell surface proteins in a single measurement is technically challenging due to a range of factors, including the varying affinities of antibodies in use, and the currently limited range of suitable fluorophores for multicolor flow cytometry measurements. Thus, it is not currently feasible to test all available antibodies against suspected cell surface proteins on one particular cell type in order to generate a more global view of the cell surface protein landscape and the development of immunoassays for additional proteins is slow and tedious.

We have developed a robust, MS-based technology for the multiplexed identification and quantification of cell surface glycoproteins and their N-glycosites. The CSC method provides a more comprehensive and more specific view of the cell surface protein landscape compared to prior methods, and circumvents the issues and limitations cited above to a large extent. This CSC approach takes advantage of a common, distinguishing feature of most cell surface proteins, i.e. the fact that they are glycosylated. By selective chemical tagging of the cell surface polysaccharides, as they are presented on the surface of live cells, we have been able to exclusively target the pool of cell surface-expressed glycoproteins for subsequent, in depth analysis, using conventional quantitative proteomic technologies.

To achieve the desired high specificity for cell surface glycopeptides, we used a gentle, multi-step chemical tagging approach for covalently labeling glycoproteins via their extracellular glycan moieties. This chemistry works for essentially all modes of protein glycosylation. This is in contrast to the use of lectins, which isolate subsets of the glyco-proteome based on their respective substrate specificity. The CSC data generated from insect cells where sialic acid residues cannot be detected, as well as the Neuraminidase experiment confirm that the sodium periodate concentrations used within the CSC experiments enabled glycoprotein labeling and that CSC technology is not dependent on terminal silac acid residues for glycoprotein identification[38, 43-46]. However, in the Neuraminidase control experiment we could observe a slight decrease in redundant peptide observations due to less total ion current (TIC) signal intensity from the N-glycosites. This is to be expected since we loose the TIC signal which would result from the additional capturing and release from formerly sialylated glycopeptides. The insect cell data also shows that the CSC technology enables the identification of the cell surface glyco-proteome in

3.6 Discussion

an organism where almost no antibodies exist to detect these cell surface glycoproteins. Also, while affinity-based or subcellular fractionation-based methods for isolating cell surface proteins are confounded by co-isolation on non-cell surface (membrane) proteins, the high specificity and selectivity obtained by CSC, through the combination of live cell labeling, avidin-affinity peptide enrichment and PNGase F cleavage of N-glyosylation modifications, allow us, for the first time, to assert with high confidence that the identified proteins are *bona fide* cell surface proteins. Additionally, by using spectrometers with sufficient mass resolution to clearly distinguish between asparagine and deamidated asparagine (±0.984 Da), we could directly confirm the physiological sites of N-glycosylation on the identified peptides/proteins, also with high confidence. However, the CSC technology does not allow us to make statements about potential N-glycosites that were not detected.

We have also discovered some additional benefits from the high confidence we can ascribe to both the N-glycosylation sites identified and confirmation of their extracellular orientation, when using CSC. Firstly, confirmed extracellular protein N-glycosylation sites from our CSC studies are now being tested, in combination with protein transmembrane prediction algorithms, as restrictive parameters for greatly improved prediction of the orientation of glycoproteins in the plasma membrane. Secondly, *in silico* protein folding algorithms such as Robetta[47] can similarly use information about confirmed N-glycosites as restrictive parameters for modeling protein structure since the N-glycosites must be on the surface of the computed three-dimensional protein model. Lastly, identified cell surface glycopeptides can be used as target sequences for antibody generation (US Patent 066661-0148, Methods for Characterizing Glycoproteins and Generating Antibodies for Same) again due to the fact that the identified glycopeptide sequences are necessarily on the surface of the native glycoprotein, and therefore likely accessible to soluble antibodies.

The CSC technology allows, for the first time, a more comprehensive view of the cell surface protein landscape in qualitative and quantitative terms than has previously been possible. By restricting proteomic analyses solely to the cell membrane, we can map the surface glycoproteins in an unprecedented and unbiased way. Therefore, CSC technology enables broad-based phenotyping of cells without antibodies. The glycoproteins identified represent a wide range of protein classes, which can now be observed in a rapid and multiplexed fashion, with or without perturbation or other alteration of the cell system under investigation. Without *a priori* knowledge, the CSC technology thus enables the identification of new and unknown proteins relevant to the system under study, as well as the identification of known proteins whose signaling involvement may not have been predicted from existing data. As shown above (Figure 3.7 and Supplementary Table S3.4), more than 47 known CD proteins could be observed, and relatively quantified in a single experiment. While these proteins could be

3 - Cell surface capturing of N-linked glycoproteins 63

potentially observed with antibodies too, it would take several separate analyses to screen cells with all 47 antibodies. In addition, the 72 non-CD proteins also identified in the same CSC experiment may represent new cell surface protein identifications for this particular cell type, many of which likely cannot be otherwise measured due to a lack of suitable antibody reagents for cell screening. Thus, due to the limited bandwidth provided by antibody-based characterization of cell type, most such characterizations are made on the basis of only a few known cell surface markers. We therefore think that CSC technology will allow the identification of a wide range of cell surface proteins, representing a unique pattern for each cell type, analogous to a broader cell surface protein 'barcode'. This barcode, which could be established from homogenous cell populations, would contain information about the predominant cell surface expressed proteins, as well as their relative abundance. CSC technology could thus be used to compare various cell types and states, based on their unique cell surface barcodes, and thus phenotype them without the use of or initial need for antibodies. We expect that phenotyping cells in this way could be an especially useful approach in discovery-driven clinical experiments for the detection of cell surface, disease-related, differentiation markers or potential therapeutic targets.

The CSC method is a robust, enabling technology, which can be integrated and combined with various experimental workflows. It is ideally suited for multiplexed, discovery-driven identification and quantification of cell surface glycoproteins. The dynamic range of the CSC technology and of glycoproteins which can be measured in a single experiment is restricted by the currently available MS instrumentation and is around 4-5 orders of magnitude. A limitation for the current implementation of CSC is the relatively high number of cells ($\sim 5 \times 10^7$) needed to detect the wide range of high and low abundant cell surface proteins simultaneously via MS. Another limitation is that CSC necessarily reveals an average view of the cell surface glyco-proteome over the measured cells. In contrast, antibody based methods, such as flow cytometry or immunohistochemistry, have the sensitivity to analyze single cells. We see IHC, FACS and CSC technology as complementary technologies on different levels which can profit from each other in order to reveal cell surface protein signaling landscapes and networks. With continued optimization of CSC technology, in combination with the predicted development of MS hardware and Selected Reaction Monitoring (SRM) strategies we can expect CSC to become even more useful for smaller and smaller cell populations, though single cell proteomics is maybe some way off in the distance at this point.

Like with many other new technologies, CSC opens up new questions and avenues of investigation for study. For example, how many proteins are actually expressed at the cell surface? Which of these are potential drug targets? How many different cell types, differentiable by molecular patterns, actually exist, and what new information can we glean by applying CSC technology to lesser-studied cell systems, such as cells of the nervous system or stem cells? In a new avenue of investigation, cell surface glycoprotein barcodes could be measured at different time points, for example during cellular activation and differentiation, in order to establish quantitative data points for the modeling and prediction of cellular processes, perhaps in combination with other -omics technologies such as genomics and transcriptomics. Finally, for us, cell surface proteins barcodes represent a pre-requisite for systems biology research. Currently, we are using CSC to establish a quantitative cell surface protein atlas. Such an atlas would represent a new systems biology resource for targeted CSC multiple reaction monitoring experiments. We therefore hope that new CSC users will be willing to share their data, as part of a common, and mutually beneficial effort to unravel cell surface signaling networks on a global scale.

3.7 References

1. Wollscheid, B. et al. Mass-spectrometric identification and relative quantification of N-linked cell surface glycoproteins. *Nat Biotechnol* **27**, 378-86 (2009).
2. Von Heijne, G. The membrane protein universe: what's out there and why bother? *J Intern Med* **261**, 543-57 (2007).
3. Wollscheid, B. et al. Lipid raft proteins and their identification in T lymphocytes. *Subcell Biochem* **37**, 121-52 (2004).
4. Hosen, N. et al. CD96 is a leukemic stem cell-specific marker in human acute myeloid leukemia. *Proc Natl Acad Sci USA* **104**, 11008-13 (2007).
5. Hopkins, A.L. & Groom, C.R. The druggable genome. *Nature reviews Drug discovery* **1**, 727-30 (2002).
6. Stewart, C.C. & Stewart, S.J. Immunophenotyping. *Current protocols in cytometry / editorial board, J Paul Robinson, managing editor [et al]* **Chapter 6**, Unit 6.2 (2001).
7. Zola, H. et al. CD molecules 2006--human cell differentiation molecules. *J Immunol Methods* **319**, 1-5 (2007).
8. Zola, H. Medical applications of leukocyte surface molecules--the CD molecules. *Mol Med* **12**, 312-6 (2006).
9. Ahram, M., Litou, Z.I., Fang, R. & Al-Tawallbeh, G. Estimation of membrane proteins in the human proteome. *In Silico Biol (Gedrukt)* **6**, 379-86 (2006).
10. Nicholson, I.C., Ayhan, M., Hoogenraad, N.J. & Zola, H. In silico evaluation of two mass spectrometry-based approaches for the identification of novel human leukocyte cell-surface proteins. *J Leukoc Biol* **77**, 190-8 (2005).
11. Craig, F.E. & Foon, K.A. Flow cytometric immunophenotyping for hematologic neoplasms. *Blood* **111**, 3941-67 (2008).
12. Evans, E.J. et al. The T cell surface--how well do we know it? *Immunity* **19**, 213-23 (2003).
13. Aebersold, R.H. & Mann, M. Mass spectrometry-based proteomics. *Nature* **422**, 198-207 (2003).
14. Bantscheff, M., Schirle, M., Sweetman, G., Rick, J. & Kuster, B. Quantitative mass spectrometry in proteomics: a critical review. *Analytical and bioanalytical chemistry* **389**, 1017-31 (2007).
15. Macher, B.A. & Yen, T.Y. Proteins at membrane surfaces-a review of approaches. *Mol Biosyst* **3**, 705-13 (2007).
16. Josic, D. & Clifton, J.G. Mammalian plasma membrane proteomics. *Proteomics* **7**, 3010-29 (2007).
17. Pasini, E.M. et al. In-depth analysis of the membrane and cytosolic proteome of red blood cells. *Blood* **108**, 791-801 (2006).
18. Andersen, J.S. & Mann, M. Organellar proteomics: turning inventories into insights. *EMBO Rep* **7**, 874-9 (2006).
19. Han, D.K., Eng, J.K., Zhou, H. & Aebersold, R.H. Quantitative profiling of differentiation-induced microsomal proteins using isotope-coded affinity tags and mass spectrometry. *Nat Biotechnol* **19**, 946-51 (2001).
20. Nunomura, K. et al. Cell surface labeling and mass spectrometry reveal diversity of cell surface markers and signaling molecules expressed in undifferentiated mouse embryonic stem cells. *Mol Cell Proteomics* **4**, 1968-76 (2005).
21. Rybak, J.N. et al. In vivo protein biotinylation for identification of organ-specific antigens accessible from the vasculature. *Nat Methods* **2**, 291-8 (2005).
22. Zhang, W., Zhou, G., Zhao, Y., White, M.A. & Zhao, Y. Affinity enrichment of plasma membrane for proteomics analysis. *Electrophoresis* **24**, 2855-63 (2003).
23. Arnott, D. et al. Selective detection of membrane proteins without antibodies: a mass spectrometric version of the Western blot. *Mol Cell Proteomics* **1**, 148-56 (2002).
24. Lewandrowski, U., Moebius, J., Walter, U. & Sickmann, A. Elucidation of N-glycosylation sites on human platelet proteins: a glycoproteomic approach. *Mol Cell Proteomics* **5**, 226-33 (2006).

25. Kaji, H., Yamauchi, Y., Takahashi, N. & Isobe, T. Mass spectrometric identification of N-linked glycopeptides using lectin-mediated affinity capture and glycosylation site-specific stable isotope tagging. *Nat Protoc* **1**, 3019-27 (2006).
26. Wu, C.C., MacCoss, M.J., Howell, K.E. & Yates, J.R. A method for the comprehensive proteomic analysis of membrane proteins. *Nat Biotechnol* **21**, 532-8 (2003).
27. Elortza, F. et al. Proteomic analysis of glycosylphosphatidylinositol-anchored membrane proteins. *Mol Cell Proteomics* **2**, 1261-70 (2003).
28. Watarai, H. et al. Plasma membrane-focused proteomics: dramatic changes in surface expression during the maturation of human dendritic cells. *Proteomics* **5**, 4001-11 (2005).
29. Zhang, H., Li, X.J., Martin, D.B. & Aebersold, R.H. Identification and quantification of N-linked glycoproteins using hydrazide chemistry, stable isotope labeling and mass spectrometry. *Nat Biotechnol* **21**, 660-6 (2003).
30. Varki, A. et al. Essentials of Glycobiology (2002).
31. Kim, J.E. & White, F.M. Quantitative analysis of phosphotyrosine signaling networks triggered by CD3 and CD28 costimulation in Jurkat cells. *J Immunol* **176**, 2833-43 (2006).
32. Bayer, E.A., Ben-Hur, H. & Wilchek, M. Biocytin hydrazide--a selective label for sialic acids, galactose, and other sugars in glycoconjugates using avidin-biotin technology. *Anal Biochem* **170**, 271-81 (1988).
33. Gahmberg, C.G. & Andersson, L.C. Selective radioactive labeling of cell surface sialoglycoproteins by periodate-tritiated borohydride. *J Biol Chem* **252**, 5888-94 (1977).
34. Yates, J.R., Eng, J.K. & McCormack, A.L. Mining genomes: correlating tandem mass spectra of modified and unmodified peptides to sequences in nucleotide databases. *Anal Chem* **67**, 3202-10 (1995).
35. Keller, A., Nesvizhskii, A.I., Kolker, E. & Aebersold, R.H. Empirical statistical model to estimate the accuracy of peptide identifications made by MS/MS and database search. *Anal Chem* **74**, 5383-92 (2002).
36. Nesvizhskii, A.I., Keller, A., Kolker, E. & Aebersold, R.H. A statistical model for identifying proteins by tandem mass spectrometry. *Anal Chem* **75**, 4646-58 (2003).
37. Shannon, P. et al. Cytoscape: a software environment for integrated models of biomolecular interaction networks. *Genome Res* **13**, 2498-504 (2003).
38. North, S.J. et al. Glycomic studies of Drosophila melanogaster embryos. *Glycoconj J* **23**, 345-54 (2006).
39. Thomas, P.D. et al. PANTHER: a browsable database of gene products organized by biological function, using curated protein family and subfamily classification. *Nucleic Acids Res* **31**, 334-41 (2003).
40. Krogh, A., Larsson, B., Von Heijne, G. & Sonnhammer, E.L. Predicting transmembrane protein topology with a hidden Markov model: application to complete genomes. *J Mol Biol* **305**, 567-80 (2001).
41. Schamel, W.W. & Reth, M. Monomeric and oligomeric complexes of the B cell antigen receptor. *Immunity* **13**, 5-14 (2000).
42. Sancho, D., Gómez, M. & Sánchez-Madrid, F. CD69 is an immunoregulatory molecule induced following activation. *Trends Immunol* **26**, 136-40 (2005).
43. Schiess, R. et al. Analysis of cell surface proteome changes via label-free, quantitative mass spectrometry. *Mol Cell Proteomics* **8**, 624-38 (2009).
44. Jarvis, D.L. Developing baculovirus-insect cell expression systems for humanized recombinant glycoprotein production. *Virology* **310**, 1-7 (2003).
45. Aumiller, J.J., Hollister, J.R. & Jarvis, D.L. A transgenic insect cell line engineered to produce CMP-sialic acid and sialylated glycoproteins. *Glycobiology* **13**, 497-507 (2003).
46. Viswanathan, K. et al. Engineering sialic acid synthetic ability into insect cells: identifying metabolic bottlenecks and devising strategies to overcome them. *Biochemistry* **42**, 15215-25 (2003).
47. Chivian, D. et al. Automated prediction of CASP-5 structures using the Robetta server. *Proteins* **53 Suppl 6**, 524-33 (2003).

4 Analysis of cell surface proteome changes via label-free, quantitative mass spectrometry

4.1 Authorship

The analysis of cell surface proteome changes via label-free, quantitative mass spectrometry comprised a main part of my Ph.D. work. Our biomarker concept relies on the assumption that the abundance level of glycoproteins secreted, shed or otherwise released by the cells reflects the disease state of tissue and organs. In order to test this hypothesis I developed a quantitative method for the analysis of cell surface glycoproteins and showed that indeed the cell surface proteome mirrors changes occurring within the cell. The findings in this study indicate that the systematic analysis of this important subproteome opens the possibility of detecting molecular signatures in body fluids and therefore is of interest for the wide field of biomarker discovery. The work is shared with Lukas Müller, Alexander Schmidt, Markus Müller, Bernd Wollscheid and Ruedi Aebersold who helped with the experimental design and the MS analysis. I also thank Martin Jünger and Matthias Gstaiger for helpful discussions and James Sorrel Eddes for bioinformatics support. This chapter represents the reformatted research article from *Molecular & Cellular Proteomics* (Schiess, R. et al., *Mol Cell Proteomics* **8**, 624-38 (2009)[1])

4.2 Summary

We present a mass spectrometry-based strategy for the specific detection and quantification of cell surface proteome changes. The method is based on the label-free quantification of peptide patterns acquired by high mass accuracy mass spectrometry using new software tools, and the Cell Surface Capturing (CSC) technology that selectively enriches glycopeptides exposed to the cell exterior. The method was applied to monitor dynamic protein changes in the cell surface glyco-proteome of *Drosophila melanogaster* cells. The results led to the construction of a cell surface glycoprotein atlas consisting of 202 cell surface glycoproteins of *D. melanogaster* Kc167 cells, and indicated relative quantitative changes of cell surface glycoproteins in four different cellular states. Furthermore, we specifically investigated cell surface proteome changes upon prolonged insulin stimulation. The data revealed insulin-dependent cell surface glycoprotein dynamics, including insulin receptor internalization, and linked these changes to intracellular signaling networks.

4.3 Introduction

The multitude of cells and cell types that constitute multicellular organisms are organized in intricate higher order structures and organs. These cells also communicate with each other, either via direct cell-to-cell contact or, over longer distances, via soluble mediators. In either form of communication the proteins at the surface of the cell, including adhesion molecules, channel transporter proteins, cell surface receptors and enzymes are of critical importance for sensing, inducing and catalyzing responses to the cell's changing environment. The ensemble of cell surface proteins, the cell surface proteome, therefore provides a unique molecular fingerprint to classify cells and cellular states. For these reasons, there has been considerable interest in a robust, sensitive, specific and quantitative technology to study the cell surface proteome.

Mass spectrometry (MS) is the method of choice for the identification and accurate quantification of the proteins contained in complex sample mixtures[2]. Recent advances in MS based proteomics, specifically improved instrumentation, software tools for the analysis of proteomic data sets[3] and emerging, more efficient data collection strategies[4], now routinely lead to the identification of hundreds to thousands of proteins in a single experiment. However, they still fall short of complete proteome analysis. As an alternative to the analysis of total cell or tissue extracts which lead to the identification and, if suitable quantification strategies are applied[5], also to the quantification of a fraction of the proteins present in the sample, it has been suggested to analyze specific subproteomes that are enriched for proteins of particular types[6]. Implementations of this concept so far include the selective isolation and subsequent analysis of cysteine containing peptides[7], phosphorylated peptides[8], N-glycosylated peptides[9], the set of N-terminal peptides[10] and specific subcellular fractions and organelles[11, 12]. These enrichment technologies have in common that a particular subset of proteins or peptides is enriched and can be analyzed more comprehensively, so that even low abundant proteins can potentially be detected.

Traditionally, cells have often been classified by exploiting antibodies available for a limited number of molecules termed clusters of differentiation (CD)[13]. These antibodies also provide a powerful tool to investigate expression changes of CD molecules and are widely used in the fields of hematology, immunology and pathology for research, diagnosis and therapy. However, the generation and validation of such monoclonal antibodies is time consuming, labor intensive and associated with high costs. Moreover, many cell types and disease states cannot be unambiguously identified with the currently available set of CD molecules. Thus, clinical and basic biology research would greatly benefit from a broader selection of such differentiation markers. In the absence of a broader set of CD specific reagents or a different approach to measure cell surface proteins more comprehensively, the characterization of this important class of proteins will remain incomplete and biased.

4 - Label-free quantitative cell surface proteomics

In contrast to the human and murine species, where at least a subset of the cell surface proteins can be detected and quantified using the anti-CD antibodies, these critical reagents are almost completely lacking for organisms such as *D. melanogaster* or *C. elegans*. However, extensive high quality data sets on proteomes or subproteomes are particularly useful in those species because they can be related to the readily accessible rich genomic and genetic resources. In prior work we have extensively mapped out the proteome and phospho-proteome of *D. melanogaster*[14, 15] and efforts by others have elucidated the metabolic protein network in the fly[16]. In combination, these resources help to position this species for integrative studies in the emerging systems biology paradigm.

In spite of the obvious interest in the cell surface proteome, technical limitations have so far precluded its comprehensive analysis. These include difficulties in efficiently separating membrane-associated from other cellular proteins, their frequently low abundance and poor solubility[17]. To facilitate the deep and specific analysis of cell surface proteins we recently developed a method for the selective identification of cell surface glycoproteins – the Cell Surface Capturing (CSC) method[18]. CSC is based on the fact that the majority of proteins on the surface of cells are glycosylated[19]. It comprises a highly selective procedure to enrich for the *N*-glycosylated peptides from glycoproteins via chemical reactivity of their carbohydrate moiety[9]. By analyzing only the *N*-glycosites (peptides that are *N*-glycosylated in the intact protein, in their de-glycosylated form), the sample complexity is drastically reduced and a relatively large abundance range of the cell surface proteome can be analyzed by mass spectrometry without the need for multidimensional separation. Therefore CSC represents a valuable tool to generate a comprehensive cell surface map in a single LC-MS analysis.

In this study we used the CSC method to characterize the cell surface proteome of the *D. melanogaster* Kc167 cell line and, in combination with label-free quantitative MS, to determine perturbation-induced changes in the surface proteome of the cell. Label-free quantification was achieved by comparing LC-MS feature maps using the software tool *SuperHirn*[20] and a new interactive software tool called *JRatio* with a GUI for the relative protein quantification of MS1 features detected in the different patterns. These experiments resulted in the identification of 202 glycoproteins 183 (91%) of which contained at least one transmembrane (TM) domain. We determined that the variation of biological replicates was below 25%, which allowed to distinguish between different cellular states based on the cell surface protein patterns consisting of *N*-glycosites representing more than a hundred glycoproteins. Upon perturbation of specific pathways within the cell, quantitative analysis revealed abundance changes in the surface glycoproteome. Furthermore, we monitored the internalization of the insulin receptor (InR) upon prolonged insulin stimulation[21] and thereby confirmed the down-regulation of the InR from the cell surface.

Additionally, we demonstrated that this change was due to InR internalization into endosomes and not degradation.

In conclusion, the work presented here describes a robust, sensitive, specific and quantitative method to profile cell surface proteomes. Its application is well suited to monitoring quantitative protein changes in multiple samples and thus has the potential to facilitate initial biomarker discovery.

4.4 Experimental Procedures

Chemicals. Porcine trypsin, modified, sequencing grade, was purchased from Promega (Madison, WI, USA). Tris(2-carboxyethyl)phosphine (TCEP) and iodoacetamide were purchased from Fluka (Buchs, Switzerland). HPLC-grade water and acetonitrile were purchased from Riedel-de Haën (Seelze, Germany), sodium periodate (Pierce), biocytin hydrazide (Biotium), UltraLink immobilized Streptavidin PLUS (Pierce), 15 ml Dounce Tissue Grinder (Wheaton, USA), RapiGest (Waters), PNGase F (NEB), Affi-Prep Hz Hydrazide (BioRad).

Cell culture. *D. melanogaster* embryonic Kc167 cells were maintained as described elsewhere[22]. Briefly, *D. melanogaster* Kc167 cells were maintained at 25°C in Schneider's *D. melanogaster* medium (Gibco/Invitrogen) supplemented with 10% heat-inactivated fetal bovine serum, FBS, 100 U/ml penicillin and 100 µg/ml streptomycin. Cells were first seeded in flasks at 5×10^6 cells/ml in a volume of 40 ml and were sub cultured every third or fourth day. Then, 80 ml of Kc167 was diluted 1:3 in an Erlenmeyer flask. Cells were harvested at OD_{600} 0.5-0.6.

Stimulation of Kc167 cells. Cells were incubated in Schneider's *D. melanogaster* medium with either 1 µg/ml lipopoly-saccharide (Sigma), 50 nM rapamycin (LC Laboratories, USA), or 1 mM sodium-vanadate (Sigma) (all final concentrations) for 1 h. Persistent insulin stimulation was achieved by first starving the cells in serum free Schneider's medium over night and then incubating them with 100 nM bovine insulin (Sigma) for 2 h.

Cell Surface Capturing (CSC). Cell Surface Capturing was performed as described by B. Wollscheid et al.[18]. *D. melanogaster* Kc167 cells were harvested by spinning them down at 450 rcf for 5 min in a centrifuge. Then, the cells were reconstituted in labeling buffer (1x PBS, 0.1% FBS, pH 6.5) and oxidized with 1.25 mM sodium periodate for 15 min at room temperature. Cells were then washed twice with labeling buffer to remove dead cells and sodium periodate. The cells were afterwards incubated with 25 mg/ml biocytin hydrazide (Biotium) to label the oxidized carbohydrates of the cell surface molecules with biotin. Biotin-labeled cells were lysed in detergent free lysis buffer (10 mM Tris-HCL, 0.5 mM

4 - Label-free quantitative cell surface proteomics

MgCl$_2$, pH 7.5) at 4°C for 10 min. Then, the cells were additionally homogenized with 30 strokes using a Dounce Tissue Grinder (Wheaton, USA). Cell debris and nuclei were removed by centrifugation at 2'800 rcf for 10 min and membranes were pelleted from the supernatant by ultracentrifugation at 210'000 rcf for 1 h. The membrane fraction was solubilized with 0.1% RapiGest (Waters) in 100 mM ammonium bicarbonate. After reduction of disulfide bonds with 5 mM TCEP for 30 min at 37°C and alkylation of cysteines with 10 mM iodoacetamide 30 min at room temperature, the proteins were digested with trypsin at an enzyme to protein ratio of 1:100 at 37°C overnight. 400 µl of a 50% slurry of UltraLink immobilized Streptavidin PLUS beads in 100 mM ammonium bicarbonate was added to the protein digest and incubated for 1 h in a head over head shaker at room teperature. Unbound peptides and lipids were then washed away with various buffers (5 M NaCl, 0.5% Triton in PBS pH 8.0, 100 mM sodium carbonate pH 11.0) followed by the specific release of N-glycosites by PNGase F (NEB) in 50 mM ammonium bicarbonate pH 7.8 at 37°C overnight. Released N-glycosites were dried in a speed vac concentrator and re-solubilized in 0.1% formic acid for mass spectrometric analysis.

Whole membrane glycocapturing. Glycoproteins were enriched from cell culture using a modified version of the protocol published by H. Zhang et al.[9]. *D. melanogaster* Kc167 cells were harvested by spinning them down at 450 rcf for 5 min in a centrifuge. The cells were lysed in detergent free lysis buffer (10 mM Tris-HCL, 0.5 mM MgCl$_2$, pH 7.5) at 4°C for 10 min. Then, the cells were additionally homogenized with 30 strokes using a Dounce Tissue Grinder (Wheaton, USA). Cell debris and nuclei were removed by centrifugation at 2'800 rcf for 10 min and membranes were pelleted from the supernatant by ultracentrifugation at 210'000 rcf for 1 h. The membrane fraction was solubilized with 0.1% RapiGest in 100 mM ammonium bicarbonate. After reduction of disulfide bonds with 5 mM TCEP for 30 min at 37°C and alkylation of cysteines with 10 mM iodoacetamide 30 min at room temperature, the proteins were digested with trypsin at an enzyme to protein ratio of 1:100 at 37°C overnight. The peptides were cleaned by reversed phase chromatography, oxidized with 20 mM sodium periodate and coupled to Affi-Prep Hz hydrazide support (BioRad). Unbound peptides and lipids were then washed away with various buffers (1.5 M NaCl, pure methanol, 80% acetonitrile, 50 mM ammonium bicarbonate) followed by the specific release of N-glycosites by PNGase F in 50 mM ammonium bicarbonate pH 7.8 at 37°C overnight. Released N-glycosites were dried in a speed vac concentrator and re-solubilized in 0.1% formic acid for mass spectrometric analysis.

Isotopic labeling. Isotopic labeling was carried out as described by Schmidt et al.[23]. The membrane protein fractions were prepared and biotin labeled as described above and proteolized. The resulting peptides were labeled with either the heavy or the light version of the ICPL reagent, respectively and the biotinylated glycopeptides were then specifically enriched as described above.

4.4 Experimental Procedures

Mass spectrometry. Samples were analyzed on a hybrid LTQ-FT mass spectrometer (Thermo Electron, San Jose, CA) equipped with a nanoelectrospray ion source. Chromatographic separation of peptides was performed on an Agilent 1100 micro HPLC system (Waldbronn, Germany), equipped with a 15 cm fused silica emitter, 150 μm inner diameter, packed with a Magic C18 AQ 5 μm resin (Michrom BioResources, Auburn, CA, USA). Peptides were loaded on the column from a cooled (4°C) Agilent autosampler and separated with a linear gradient of acetonitrile/water, containing 0.1% formic acid, at a flow rate of 1.2 μl/min. A linear gradient from 2 to 28% acetonitrile in 60 min which was optimized for the number of peptide features detected was used. The MS instrument was operated to maximize the quality of LC-MS feature maps as opposed to maximizing the number of identifications. Therefore, for each peptide sample a standard data-dependent acquisition (DDA) on the three most intense ions per MS-scan was performed. Three MS/MS spectra were acquired in the linear ion trap per FT-MS scan, the latter acquired at 100'000 FWHM (at 350 m/z) nominal resolution, resulting in an overall cycle time of approximately 1 second. Charge state screening was employed, allowing fragmentation of doubly and higher charged ions, and rejecting ions of single and unknown charge state. A threshold of 200 ion counts was set to trigger an MS/MS attempt.

Data analysis. The raw data acquired by the LTQ-FT (software: Xcalibur 2.0 SR1) was converted to mzXML using ReAdW 3.5.1[24] applying default parameters. MS/MS scans were then exported as .dta files without further processing using the program mzXML2Other[24]. MS/MS spectra were searched against the Berkeley *D. melanogaster* Genome Project BDGP5.2 (20'981 entries) database using SEQUEST v.27[25]. The SEQUEST database search criteria included variable modifications of 57.02146 Da for cysteines (for the alkylation with iodoacetamide in order to combine search results of both reduced/alkylated and non-reduced/non-alkylated samples), 15.99491 Da for methionines (for oxidation), and of 0.98406 Da for potential formerly *N*-glycosylated asparagines (which are converted to aspartic acid by PNGase F release), respectively. The following additional search constraints were applied: monoisotopic parent and fragment masses, precursor-ion mass tolerance: 0.05 Da, fragment-ion mass tolerance 0.5 Da, at least 1 tryptic terminus, 1 missed cleavage. The identified peptides were processed and analyzed through the mass spectrometry Trans-Proteomic Pipeline 3.5 (TPP)[26]. In the TPP, the database search results were validated using the PeptideProphet software[27], which uses various SEQUEST scores (XCorr, ΔC_n, SpRank) to calculate a probability score for each identified peptide by linear discriminant analysis. *N*-glycosylation motif information and accurate mass binning were used in PeptideProphet. The peptides were then assigned for protein identification using the ProteinProphet software[28]. ProteinProphet allowed filtering of large-scale data sets with assessment of predictable sensitivity and false positive identification error rates. In this study, we used a PeptideProphet probability score ≥ 0.9, and a ProteinProphet

4 - Label-free quantitative cell surface proteomics

probability score ≥ 0.9. This resulted in an overall false positive error rate below 1% as determined by ProteinProphet[28].

For the quantitation of the ICPL differential labeling experiment, the XPRESS software integrated in the TPP was used[29]. Protein ratios were calculated by accurately quantifying the relative abundance of ICPL-labeled peptides from their chromatographic co-elution profiles. Starting with the peptide identification, XPRESS isolates d0 and d4 peptide elution profiles, determines the area of each peptide peak, and calculates the abundance ratio based on these areas.

Transmembrane prediction. Transmembrane domain predictions were obtained from the SOSUI web server (http://sosui.proteome.bio.tuat.ac.jp/sosuiframe0E.html) for classification and secondary structure prediction of membrane proteins[30] and TMHMM, a hidden Markov model based predictor for transmembrane helices in protein sequences[31].

Label-free quantification of peptide and protein ratios. Data from LC-MS runs were converted from raw to the mzXML data format[24] and processed by the software tool SuperHirn (http://tools.proteomecenter.org/SuperHirn.php)[20]. SuperHirn performs feature detection on acquired LC-MS feature maps whereby isotopic patterns of peptides are extracted and tracked along their chromatographic elution profile. It centroids raw peak data and reduces m/z signals of an MS1 scan to the corresponding monoisotopic masses, along with the charge state (z). The integrated peak area of the detected MS1 feature is calculated from the intensity values of the detected monoisotopic peak areas over the chromatographic elution period. Acquired peptide identifications in pepXML format[27] were then mapped to the extracted MS1 features via their accurate precursor mass and retention time coordinate. MS1 features are then mapped across the different LC-MS maps and integrated into a general repository of aligned MS1 features, designated MasterMap. The MasterMap represents a framework for further data analysis such as intensity normalization and the extraction of MS1 feature, peptide and protein ratios.

In order to increase the number of proteins identified, we used the inclusion list annotation feature of SuperHirn where peptide identifications from targeted MS/MS experiments can be mapped back to detected MS1 features[4]. Thereby the MasterMap was further updated with MS/MS information in order to assign MS1 features which had not been annotated in a particular experiment with the corresponding peptide sequence. The acquired peptide identifications were mapped back to corresponding MS1 features using accurate mass, normalized retention time (ΔRT = 1.0 min) and the peptide charge information[16].

The in-house developed Java software JRatio was used for the calculation and visual assessment of peptide and protein ratios. Specifically, JRatio imports aligned MS1 features from the MasterMap and quantifies fold changes of MS1 features across LC-MS measurements. In a first step, fold changes of

4.4 Experimental Procedures

aligned MS1 features were quantified by computing ratios between sample states from the average MS1 feature intensities $\overline{V}_{A/B}$ from replicate measurements of treatment group A and B, respectively (formula 1). Accordingly, standard deviations of the computed ratios were derived as described in formula 2.

$$R_{Feature\frac{A}{B}} = \frac{\overline{V}_A}{\overline{V}_B} \quad (1)$$

$$\sigma_{Feature\frac{A}{B}} = R_{Feature\frac{A}{B}} \cdot \sqrt{\left(\frac{\sigma_{V_A}}{\overline{V}_A}\right)^2 + \left(\frac{\sigma_{V_B}}{\overline{V}_B}\right)^2} \quad (2)$$

JRatio provides visual support for the assessment of the computed results where MS1 feature ratios can be explored to verify the extracted chromatographic elution profiles and intensity reproducibility of aligned MS1 features between replicate runs etc. Proteins were then assembled from MS1 feature ratios characterized by a high quality MS/MS peptide identification (PeptideProphet probability $\geq 0.9^{27}$). Importantly, only fully tryptic N-glycosites were taken into account for protein quantification. Robust protein ratios and standard deviations were derived for each protein from its associated MS1 feature ratios (Formula 3 and 4). A normal distribution was used to describe the calculated protein ratios and t-student test statistics was applied to assess the significance of a protein fold change. Proteins with a P-value smaller than 0.1 were considered to be significantly regulated. JRatio is freely available and can be downloaded from the following website: http://prottools.ethz.ch/muellelu/web/JRatio.php.

$$R_{Protein\frac{A}{B}} = \frac{\sum_{i=1}^{N_{R_{Feature}}} \frac{R_{Feature,i}}{\sqrt{\sigma_{Feature,i}}}}{\sum_{i=1}^{N_{R_{Feature}}} \frac{1}{\sqrt{\sigma_{Feature,i}}}} \quad (3)$$

$$\sigma_{Protein\frac{A}{B}} = \frac{\sqrt{\sum_{i=1}^{N_{R_{Feature}}} (\sigma_{Feature,i})^2}}{N_{R_{Feature}}} \quad (4)$$

4.5 Results

The goal of this study was to test the hypothesis that different cellular states can be distinguished by the comprehensive, fast and quantitative analysis of the cell surface proteome. We approached this by combining the selective enrichment of cell surface glycoproteins with a label-free, quantitative proteomics method that provides the sample throughput required to analyze multiple samples. To test the specificity and the sensitivity of the method, cell surface proteins in *D. melanogaster* Kc167 cells were selectively isolated and a comprehensive catalogue of 202 cell surface glycosylated proteins was generated. We then assessed the reproducibility of the label-free quantification approach. Subsequently, changes in the cell surface glyco-proteome induced by specific perturbations were quantitatively monitored, indicating that the cell surface glyco-proteome indeed changed as a function of the cell's state. Finally, we validated the technique by applying it to a well-studied biological system, the regulation of insulin receptor (InR) action.

4.5.1 The *D. melanogaster* Kc167 cell surface glyco-proteome atlas

We first identified the *N*-glycosites from the *D. melanogaster* Kc167 cell surface proteome to generate a reference map for further comparative analyses by label-free quantitative MS. The *N*-glycosites were identified by LC-MS/MS after their isolation via the Cell Surface Capturing (CSC) method that is based on selective affinity labeling and solid-phase capturing of glycosylated cell surface peptides[18]. The data were stored in a database (Kc167 glyco-proteome atlas) and are represented in a LC-MS (retention time (RT) vs. *m/z*) feature map (Figure 4.1) in which the identified *N*-glycosites were annotated with their amino acid sequence.

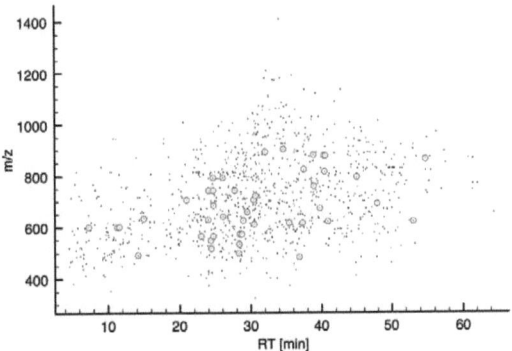

Figure 4.1 Cell surface LC-MS map of *N*-glycosites. Graphical representation of the LC-MS (retention time (RT) vs. *m/z*) feature map. Only the identified *N*-glycosites are shown. Red dots represent *N*-glycosites originating from the InR. The InR has 25 potential *N*-glycosylation sites of which 19 could be verified by the 44 *N*-glycosites described here.

4.5 Results

To generate the dataset we combined the results of 12 experiments in which cell surface glycoproteins from *D. melanogaster* Kc167 cells were isolated and subjected to LC-MS/MS. The fragment ion spectra acquired from a total of 90 LC-MS/MS runs were searched against the database BDGP5.2 (for details see methods section). A total of 20'608 MS/MS spectra were assigned at a PeptideProphet probability[27] threshold of ≥ 0.9 (FDR 1%) to peptide sequences of which 84% (17'397) matched to peptides containing the NxS/T motif, indicating the presence of a glycan at that site in the intact protein. These results indicate the high selectivity of the method for N-glycosites.

Overall, the assigned spectra represented 1'002 unique N-glycosites (PeptideProphet probability score ≥ 0.9, FDR 1%) matching to 202 unique glycoproteins (Supplementary Table S4.1). 578 different sites of N-glycosylation could be unambiguously assigned due to the mass shift caused by enzymatic deamidation at the site of glycan attachment (mass difference: 0.98604 Da). 183 (91%) of the identified cell surface glycoproteins contained at least one transmembrane (TM) domain as predicted by SOSUI, a classification and secondary structure prediction algorithm for membrane proteins[30]. 126 out of the 202 identified proteins could be GO (gene ontology) annotated using Babelomics[32] software. 108 (86%) of the GO annotated proteins belonged to the group "membrane", 7 (5%) to the group "extracellular matrix", and only 11 (9%) were annotated as "intracellular" (Figure 4.2). Interestingly, 5 out of the 11 proteins annotated as "intracellular" contain at least one predicted transmembrane domain and therefore are likely to be also constituents of the plasma membrane.

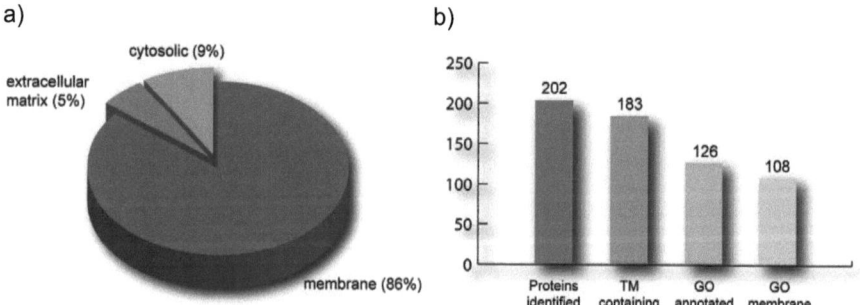

Figure 4.2 Analysis of identified cell surface glycoproteins. (a) Gene ontology (GO) cellular component analysis of the identified proteins. GO annotation for 126 proteins out of the 202 glycoproteins identified was available. 86% belonged to the membrane, 5% to the extracellular matrix, and 9% to the cytoplasm. (b) 183 out of the 202 glycoproteins identified contain one or more transmembrane (TM) domains predicted by SOSUI[30]. Furthermore 108 of the 126 GO annotated proteins are membrane constituents.

4 - Label-free quantitative cell surface proteomics

The proteins identified cover all major classes of cell-surface receptor proteins. For example, the proteins methuselah (CG6936) and methuselah-like 3 (CG6530), members of the class of the G-protein coupled receptors (GPCR) which are known to be generally of low abundance[33] were found. We also identified several enzyme-linked receptors, including the receptor tyrosine kinases InR (CG18402), Eph receptor tyrosine kinase (CG1511) and the PDGF/VEGF receptor (CG8222), as well as the membrane spanning phospho tyrosine phosphatase receptors PTP69D (CG10975), PTP10D (CG1817), and PTP4E (CG6899). Further, the cytokine receptors activin receptor (CG7904) and domeless (CG14226), the integrin adhesion molecules (CG1560, CG1771, CG8095, CG9623) that are involved in cell-cell interaction, and membrane transporters like the beta subunits 1 and 2 of the sodium/potassium-transporting ATPase (CG9258, CG9261) as well as the organic cation (CG13610) and anion transporter proteins (CG3380, CG7571) were identified. These results demonstrate that in terms of function and abundance a wide range of cell surface molecules was covered implying that our approach is neither limited to a certain subclass of cell surface proteins nor by the dynamic range.

4.5.2 Reproducible, label-free quantification of the Kc167 cell surface glyco-proteome

To assess the accuracy and reproducibility of quantifying cell surface proteome changes detected by the analysis of LC-MS maps of isolated N-glycosites, we performed biological and technical replicates of the Kc167 cell surface proteins. The CSC method was applied to cells from three parallel Kc167 cell cultures. Each of the three biological isolates was analyzed in triplicate on a high mass resolution LTQ-FT instrument. The 9 LC-MS feature maps thus generated were processed by the software SuperHirn[20]. SuperHirn identified the peptide features in each MS1 feature map and aligned them across the different maps to generate an intensity normalized MasterMap. In total, 5166 MS1 features were detected of which 1210 could be aligned over all 9 LC-MS runs. To quantify the reproducibility of the method, the coefficient of variance (CV) of feature intensity values across all 9 aligned LC-MS patterns was computed. 76% of the quantified features showed a CV equal to or below 30% and the average coefficient of variance of all 1210 aligned features was 24%. For technical replicates CVs between 10% and 13% were achieved.

Figure 4.3 illustrates the reproducibility between the biological and the technical replicates using scatter plots. In Figure 4.3a, peak intensities obtained from aligned MS1 features of three technical replicates acquired from the same biological sample were plotted against each other. The high Squared-Pearson-Correlation R^2 and the near straight lines indicated the optimal linear relationship between the replicates. Similarly, the mean peak intensities of MS1 features obtained from the three biological replicates showed very high correlation as illustrated in Figure 4.3b. Furthermore, the plots also illustrate that the intensities of the detected MS1 features span a dynamic range of more than 3 orders of magnitude.

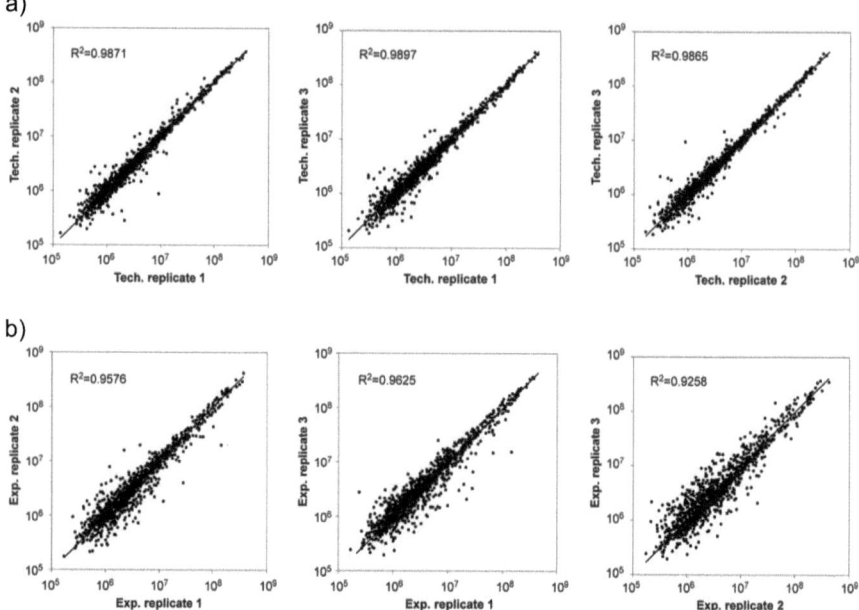

Figure 4.3 Reproducibility of label-free quantification of the Kc167 cell surface glyco-proteome. Scatter-plot of LC-MS features of isolated N-glycosites using CSC and the respective Squared-Pearson-Correlation R^2 are shown. (a) The peptide peak areas of aligned MS1 features in the 3 replicate runs of experiment 1 were plotted against each other. (b) The mean peptide peak areas of aligned MS1 features in the 3 experiments were plotted against each other.

The variation among biological experiments and their technical LC-MS replicates was further investigated by comparing the respective peak ratios. These are expected to be 1.0 because the same amount of protein was expected to be present in each sample. For each biological experiment, the average intensity of each aligned MS1 feature was calculated across the three technical replicates and then divided by the average feature intensity measured over all 9 consecutive runs belonging to the three experimental replicates. Only MS1 features detected in all 9 runs were considered for this statistical analysis. More than 95% of all MS1 feature ratios were below a 2-fold variance and 85% of all MS1 features varied by less than 40%. The same analysis was done for the three technical replicates of each experiment. 90% of the aligned MS1 features showed a ratio variation of less than 25%, which clearly demonstrates the high reproducibility of MS1 feature intensities acquired by the LTQ-FT mass spectrometer and calculated by our label-free quantification approach.

Finally, the quantification error between replicated runs of this experiment showed a variation similar to the one reported by Wang et al. in two duplicate LC-MS runs[34]. In conclusion, the combination of the method for the selective isolation of cell surface N-glycosites with label-free quantification is feasible. We demonstrate the capacity of the technique to highly enrich for the cell surface glyco-proteome and to quantify peptide features over a dynamic range of more than three orders of magnitude and for multiple samples, thus making it possible to detect and quantify even low abundance cell surface glycoproteins in serial comparisons.

4.5.3 The cell surface proteome changes as a function of cellular state

We hypothesize that the composition of the cell surface proteome reflects the state of the intracellular signaling systems and that thus perturbations in intracellular signaling systems can be detected by changes in the cell surface proteome.

To test this hypothesis Kc167 cell cultures were subjected to an array of different perturbations to induce changes in cellular state and to monitor the resulting changes in the cell surface glyco-proteome. The cells were treated either with lipopoly-saccharide (LPS) which elicits strong activation of JNK, a stress-activated protein kinase downstream of mitogen-activated protein kinases (MAPKs)[35], rapamycin, an inhibitor of the target of rapamycin (TOR) which is an important component of the insulin signaling pathway and affects cell growth by modulating the activity of S6K kinase[22], or vanadate which generally inhibits protein phosphatases and therefore triggers a whole cascade of stress-activated protein phosphorylation changes[36]. These three selected stimuli are known to have a strong effect on intracellular signaling events and thus were believed to also affect the cell surface proteome. To quantify the cell surface abundance changes introduced by the respective perturbations, each cell sample was subjected to N-glycosite enrichment and the resulting samples were analyzed on a LTQ-FT instrument and glycoprotein abundance ratios were calculated against the intensity values of an untreated control cell culture. LC-MS feature maps were analyzed as previously described and combined into a MasterMap. Additionally, MS/MS based peptide identifications of cell surface glycoproteins from the cell surface atlas were used to annotate MS1 features not sequenced in these particular LC-MS/MS runs. JRatio was then used to obtain protein ratios from MS1 features with available high quality peptide information (PeptideProphet p > 0.9) (for details see methods section).

In total, 112 N-glycosites were quantified, collectively representing 61 different glycoproteins (Supplementary Table S4.2). For each stimulus about 80% of the glycoproteins quantified showed less than 2-fold regulation. This is expected since each stimulus triggers only certain specific signaling cascades. The proteins fasciclin 1 and 2 (CG6588, CG3665), tetraspanin 86D (CG4591) and multiple integrins (CG8095, CG1771, CG1560), which are responsible for maintaining cell structure and cell adhesion and thought to have constant abundance levels, did not change at any of the conditions tested. In contrast, the glycosylated cell surface proteins guanylate cyclase (CG8742) and 26-29kD-proteinase (CG8947) showed lower, respectively higher abundance after stimulation independent of the stimulus. Other glycoproteins exhibited specific abundance changes following one or two particular stimuli. These include the macroglobulin complement-related protein (CG7586) that was up-regulated after rapamycin and vanadate treatment, a protein with similarity to the ABC transporter family (CG5789) up-regulated after vanadate treatment only and the Niemann-Pick Type C-1 protein (CG5722) that was down-regulated after LPS stimulation. The abundance ratios detected in these perturbation experiments, along with the corresponding standard deviation and P-value are shown in Table 4.1 and changes in protein abundance are illustrated with a heat map in Figure 4.4. In summary, the results illustrate that cell samples representing differentially perturbed states can be distinguished by their specific cell surface proteome patterns.

Table 4.1 Quantitative pattern of selected glycoproteins following different perturbations. The protein ratios (perturbed/non perturbed) and corresponding standard deviations (SD) including the p-values of identified and quantified glycoproteins following different perturbations. It is demonstrated that each stimuli changes abundance levels of a specific subset of cell surface glycoproteins.

Flybase ID	Annotatio nSymbol	Protein Name	LPS stimulated cell culture		Rapamycin stimulated cell culture		Vanadate stimulated cell culture		Biological process
			Protein Ratio, SD	P-val	Protein Ratio, SD	P-val	Protein Ratio, SD	P-val	
FBgn0000634	CG6588	Fasciclin 1	0.90±0.18	0.65	1.26±0.25	0.21	1.13±0.17	0.52	cell adhesion
FBgn0000635	CG3665	Fasciclin 2	0.83±0.14	0.39	1.13±0.22	0.60	1.08±0.18	0.44	cell adhesion
FBgn0003328	CG8095	Integrin alpha-PS3	1.20±0.24	0.36	1.28±0.20	0.17	1.37±0.23	0.95	cell adhesion
FBgn0004456	CG1771	Integrin alpha-PS1	0.82±0.10	0.37	0.98±0.13	0.62	1.50±0.01	0.84	cell adhesion
FBgn0004657	CG1560	Integrin beta-PS	0.95±0.04	0.85	1.17±0.32	0.45	1.32±0.04	0.86	cell adhesion
FBgn0037848	CG4591	Tetraspanin 86D	NA	NA	0.84±0.13	0.12	0.96±0.28	0.27	cell adhesion
FBgn0013974	CG8742	Guanylyl cyclase at 76C	0.36±0.17	<0.01	0.60±0.17	<0.01	0.45±0.14	<0.01	metabolic process
FBgn0028967	CG8947	26-29kD-proteinase	1.90±0.52	<0.01	2.09±0.46	<0.01	2.88±0.42	0.03	metabolic process
FBgn0039207	CG5789	CG5789	0.96±0.24	0.89	1.35±0.14	0.08	2.6±0.4	0.07	unknown
Fbgn0020240	CG7586	Macroglobulin complement-related	0.99±0.09	1.00	1.36±0.14	0.07	1.13±0.14	0.52	unknown
Fbgn0024320	CG5722	Niemann-Pick Type C-1	0.53±0.04	<0.01	0.94±0.09	0.43	0.85±0.04	0.14	multicellular organismal process

4 - Label-free quantitative cell surface proteomics

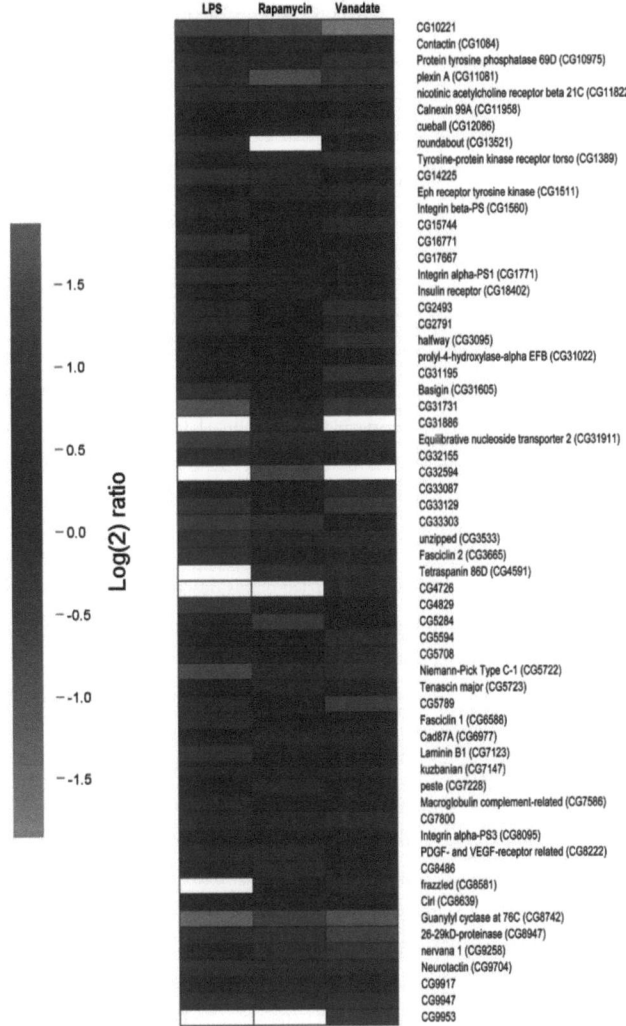

Figure 4.4 Protein abundance changes on the cell surface upon differential perturbation. Glycoproteins from different perturbation experiments are shown in color according to their log ratio from green (4-fold down-regulated) to red (4-fold up-regulated). Glycoprotein ratios were built comparing each stimulated sample to a control. White fields indicate features that were not detected or quantified in the respective sample.

4.5.4 Insulin induced internalization of Insulin Receptor (InR)

To test the ability of the described method to measure the quantitative behavior of specific cell surface proteins, we used a well-studied biological system, the regulation of the InR. Its primary function is to maintain glucose homeostasis through signaling induced by the interaction of the receptor with insulin. Signaling is modulated by reversible phosphorylation of cellular substrates, catalyzed in part by the InR tyrosine kinase and protein tyrosine phosphatases (PTPs), respectively. The InR activity is dependant on a dynamic equilibrium between surface (active) and internal (inactive) receptor pools[37]. To measure this redistribution in response to InR stimulation, Kc167 cells were starved in serum free Schneider's medium over night. Half of the cells were then incubated with 100 nM bovine insulin for 2 hours to simulate persistent insulin stimulation. Insulin stimulation was verified by pS6K western-blotting (data not shown)[38]. In parallel, the two populations of cells were subjected to the CSC method followed by the quantitative analysis of the isolated N-glycosites using the LTQ-FT instrument and subsequent comparative analysis of the LC-MS maps. The experiment was repeated to account for biological variation between experiments and 3 technical replicates were carried out and used to generate the respective MasterMaps.

Computation of peptide and protein ratios was carried out as described before. The results showed an unambiguous 2-fold down-regulation (ratio 0.41±0.07) of the InR (CG18402) that was quantified by 6 N-glycopeptides. In addition, we were able to quantify an additional 100 cell surface glycoproteins (Supplementary Table S4.3), which was about half the glycoproteins previously described in the cell surface glycoprotein atlas. We determined that the abundance of fascilin 1 (CG6588), integrins (CG8095, CG1771, CG1560) and the tetraspanins 86D and 3A (CG4591, CG10742), proteins responsible for maintaining cell structure and cell adhesion, did not change upon insulin stimulation. In contrast, some glycoproteins known to be involved in developmental processes like InR exhibited clear abundance changes. As an example, the protein frazzled (CG8581) that has netrin receptor activity and thus is involved in axon guidance[39] is 3-fold down-regulated after insulin stimulation while roundabout (CG13521), a membrane receptor with positive regulation of cell-cell adhesion is almost 3-fold up-regulated in insulin stimulated cells. Tetraspanin 42El (CG12840) is 5-fold down-regulated upon insulin stimulation. In contrast to the tetraspanins mentioned before, tetraspanin 42El is not involved in cell-cell adhesion but in developmental processes through receptor signaling. The glycoprotein changes mentioned here are summarized in Table 4.2.

4 - Label-free quantitative cell surface proteomics

Table 4.2 Quantitative pattern of selected glycoproteins following InR stimulation. Shown are the abundance ratios (insulin stimulated/non stimulated) including standard deviation (SD) and P-value of selected glycoproteins discussed here specifically that were identified and quantified upon insulin stimulation. Glycoprotein involved in cell adhesion exhibit clearly less regulation than the ones carrying out developmental processes.

Flybase ID	Protein Name	Annotation Symbol	Protein Ratio	P-value	peptides quantified	Biological process
FBgn0000634	Fasciclin 1	CG6588	0.87±0.34	0.91	7	cell adhesion
FBgn0003328	Integrin alpha-PS3	CG8095	1.20±0.58	0.38	1	cell adhesion
FBgn0004456	Integrin alpha-PS1	CG1771	1.03±0.66	0.63	1	cell adhesion
FBgn0004657	Integrin beta-PS	CG1560	0.91±0.37	0.83	4	cell adhesion
FBgn0037848	Tetraspanin 86D	CG4591	0.88±0.24	0.91	2	cell adhesion
FBgn0040334	Tetraspanin 3A	CG10742	1.05±0.39	0.59	1	cell adhesion
FBgn0013984	InR	CG18402	0.41±0.07	0.09	6	developmental process
FBgn0033134	Tetraspanin 42EI	CG12840	0.21±0.15	< 0.01	1	developmental process
FBgn0005631	roundabout	CG13521	2.73±0.68	< 0.01	1	developmental process
FBgn0011592	frazzled	CG8581	0.29±0.34	< 0.01	2	developmental process

To verify the results obtained via label-free quantification for the InR abundance changes caused by insulin treatment, we related these data obtained on parallel samples using a differential isotope labeling approach. Therefore we used half of the insulin stimulated and the control membrane fraction from the label-free quantification experiment just described before. Half of each fraction was isotopically labeled using either heavy (control) or light (insulin stimulated) isotope coded protein label (ICPL)[27]. N-glycosites were specifically enriched by CSC from the combined peptide samples as described before and analyzed twice on the LTQ-FT.

The data obtained by differential stable isotope labeling showed that the InR was 2-fold down-regulated (ratio 0.42±0.08) which confirmed the previous findings from the label-free approach (ratio 0.41±0.07). Figure 4.5 shows a MS spectrum (Figure 4.5a) as well as an elution profile (Figure 4.5b) of the glycopeptide VDLEHAN*NTESPVR originating from the InR confirming the 2-fold difference. The peptide is representative for the other 4 N-glycosites identified from the InR (Supplementary Table S4.4). The data indicate that the label-free quantification method reaches similar accuracy than that achieved by stable isotope labeling.

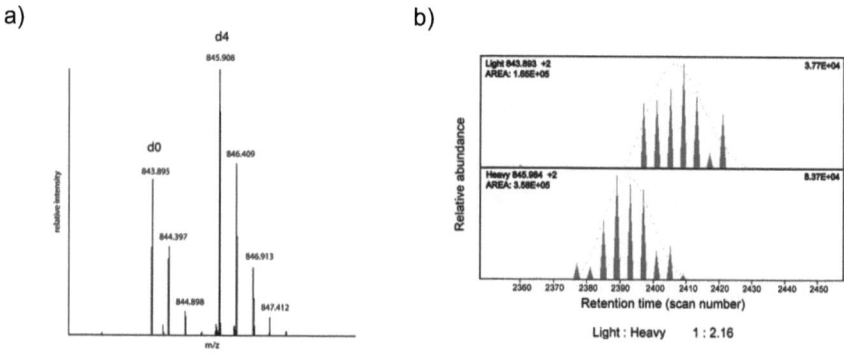

Figure 4.5 Quantitation of InR using isotope coded protein labeling. (a) MS spectra obtained over the whole elution time of VDLEHAN*NTESPVR, a formerly glycosylated peptide originating from the InR. The doubly charged species shows a lower signal for the light labeled peptide (d0 – insulin treated) than for the heavy labeled one (d4 - control). (b) Relative abundance and the calculated d0 : d4 ratio obtained using XPRESS software.

These data are in agreement with the model proposed for the regulation of InR action. Under starving conditions (in the absence of serum) and therefore in the absence of ligand, the InR accumulates at the plasma membrane. Upon insulin binding, the ligand–receptor complex is sequestered from the plasma membrane and internalized into endosomes[40]. The acidic pH of endosomes induces the dissociation of insulin from InR. While insulin is degraded by endosomal acidic insulinase[41], the InR is recycled back to the cell surface (Figure 4.6). However, under conditions of prolonged stimulation with saturating levels of insulin, a subset of the InRs are transported to the late endosome and lysosome for degradation[42].

The characteristic of the CSC method that selects for glycoproteins being present on the cells surface at the time of labeling, if related to a whole cell membrane analysis of *N*-glycosites, should allow for the differentiation of cell surface versus internalized proteins and thus for the fraction of InR being active on the cell surface and the fraction being inactivated by internalization into endosomes. To demonstrate that the InR is indeed internalized but not yet degraded, we performed a whole membrane glycocapture experiment where the cells were lysed and their membrane fraction was prepared by ultracentrifugation. From this sample we then specifically enriched for glycopeptides using a modified version of the original solid phase extraction protocol for serum glycoproteins[9]. In contrast to the CSC method where glycoproteins from the cell surface are isolated, this approach enriches for all glycoproteins present in the membrane fraction, i.e. also proteins present in membranes of internal organelles. Therefore, if the InR

4 - Label-free quantitative cell surface proteomics   85

was only internalized into vesicles but not degraded, the abundance ratio of InR measured in insulin stimulated and non-stimulated cells should not change.

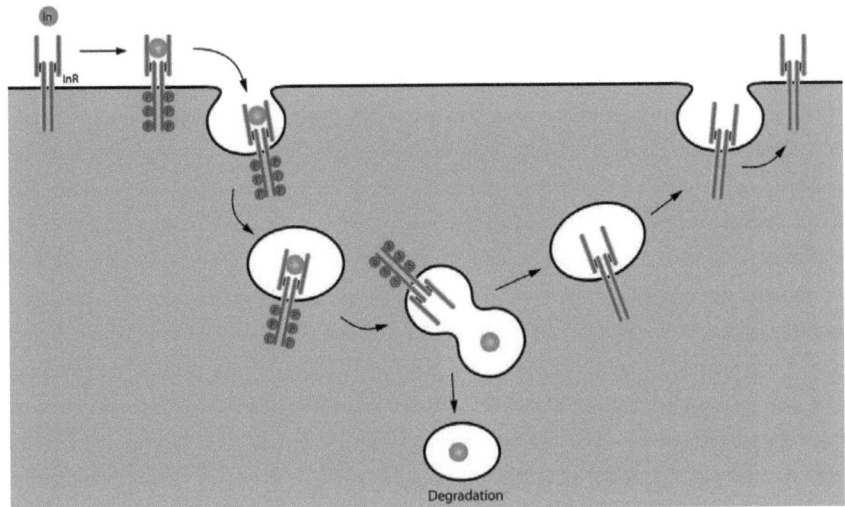

Figure 4.6 Scheme of InR recycling. Following the binding of insulin and auto-phosphorylation, InR gets internalized. After the acidification and release of insulin, InR gets de-phosphorylated and recycled back to the cell surface.

Four biological replicates of Kc167 cells were starved in serum free Schneider's medium over night followed by insulin stimulation with 100 nM bovine insulin for 2 hours for half of the cells. The two cell samples were then subjected to the whole membrane glycocapture method followed by quantitative analysis using the LTQ-FT instrument. Two technical replicates were generated for all four samples and data analysis was carried out as described before. The 132 N-glycosites identified and quantified in this experiment corresponded to 78 glycoproteins (Supplementary Table S4.5). 2 distinct N-glycosites originating from the InR were identified and quantified. The calculated abundance ratio from insulin stimulated versus non-stimulated cells was 0.94±0.24, indicating that the InR was not degraded after 2 hours of insulin stimulation. Together with the quantitative data of InR obtained by cell surface glycoprotein analysis we conclude that approximately 50% of the total receptor was compartmentalized into endosomes.

Figure 4.7 summarizes the different protein changes after insulin stimulation obtained either by the cell surface capturing or the whole membrane capturing approach. The abundance ratios of most glycoproteins observed in both analyses changed neither on the cell surface nor in the whole cell membrane. An example of this class is integrin beta-PS (CG1560) (Figure 4.7a). There were at least seven proteins, among them the protein frazzled (CG8581), tetraspanin 42 El (CG12840), a membrane spanning adenlyate cyclase (CG32158) and a potential oligosaccharyl transferase (CG1518) that were down-regulated on the cell surface while the whole membrane capturing revealed no significant abundance change, thus showing the same behavior as InR (Figure 4.7b). Another interesting pair of proteins, roundabout (CG13521) (Figure 4.7c) was up-regulated on the cell surface while the overall membrane content of these proteins was found to be constant, indicating insulin stimulated redistribution from an internal reservoir to the cell surface. The multipass membrane protein wntless (CG6210) that is specifically required for the secretion of wingless and thus participates in multiple development events, was also slightly up-regulated on the cell surface while the overall wntless protein content in the membrane decreased. The protein halfway (CG3095), involved in the antagonistic ecdysome signaling pathway, was found to be increased almost 2-fold in the whole cell membrane, however, the protein level of the same protein did not change on the cell surface, indicating insulin stimulated synthesis and storage in the cell interior. Further, NPC1 (Niemann-Pick Type C-1) protein (CG5722), involved in sterol metabolic processes, was decreased on the cell surface (0.60±0.09) as well as in the whole membrane extract (0.45±0.05) suggesting that the protein was degraded after insulin stimulation. In combination, these findings, summarized in Figure 4.7d, show that the combination of CSC and whole membrane glycocapturing enables us to study the dynamic distribution of membrane proteins after cell perturbation. In the case of insulin stimulation we observed multiple quantitative patterns for specific proteins that suggest cell internal protein redistribution, de novo synthesis and degradation.

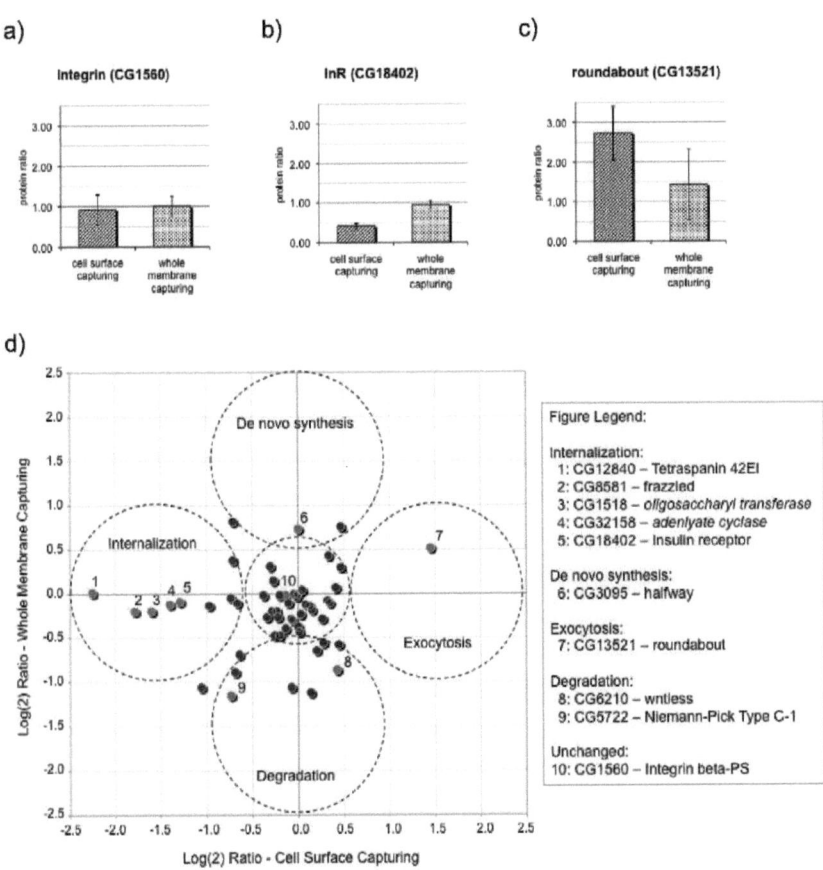

Figure 4.7 Protein abundance changes on the cell surface versus the whole cell membrane upon insulin stimulation. Protein ratios from insulin treated versus non treated cells obtained by cell surface capturing (CSC) and whole membrane capturing are shown for (a) integrin, (b) InR and (c) baboon. (d) Protein log ratios obtained from both CSC (x-axis) and whole membrane capturing (y-axis) are plotted. Only protein ratios obtained in both experiments are shown. Proteins mentioned in the text are depicted in red color. The corresponding abundance ratios of proteins quantified by both the CSC and the whole membrane capturing method are shown in bold in the Supplementary Tables S4.3 + S4.5.

4.6 Discussion

In this paper we show that the highly selective CSC method allowed for the unambiguous identification of cell surface glycoproteins in *D. melanogaster* cells, including their sites of carbohydrate linkage at a selectivity of almost 90% at the peptide level. Non-specifically isolated peptides could be readily identified due to their lack of an NxS/T glycosylation motif. This led to the identification of 202 glycoproteins from *D. melanogaster* Kc167 cells of which 91% had at least one predicted transmembrane domain and 86% of the GO annotated proteins belonging to the membrane. These results are consistent with results obtained using the same method on mammalian cells[18]. Insect cells, in contrast to mammalian cells, do not contain sialic acid which is the outermost sugar residue in mammalian carbohydrate structures and, due to its cis-diols, readily accessible for hydrazide linkage via periodate oxidation[43]. Furthermore, we have identified three peptides containing the NxC motif[44] which has not been described in insect cells to date and occurs very rarely compared to the NxS/T motif in mammalian cells. The data therefore indicate that the lack of terminal sialic acid does not limit our glycopeptide isolation strategy, a fact that extends the CSC method to other species lacking sialic acid.

To identify and quantify the isolated *N*-glycosites the samples were analyzed by ESI-MS/MS. Since one objective of the study was the quantitative comparison of the cell surface proteome of Kc167 cells in multiple perturbed states the sample throughput and accuracy of the quantitative proteomics method was a critical issue. Although quantification by spectral counting would be possible using the data obtained we decided to quantify based on the precursor intensities because it is more accurate, especially for proteins of lower abundance with few spectral counts, and is not limited to the quantification of the peptides identified by MS/MS. Moreover, we chose to explore label-free quantification via feature pattern matching because this gave us the flexibility to compare any pattern with any other pattern acquired in the context of the study. This is unlike the situation in studies depending on stable isotope labeling where the samples to be compared have to be anticipated during the design of the study. Initially, we compared the performance of isotope coded protein labels (ICPL) and label-free quantification, whereby we evaluated the relative errors arising from the biological (difference between different biological isolates) and technical (difference caused by repeat analyses of identical samples). The data indicated that the observed protein abundance changes of the two methods were very similar and, consistent with this notion, that the major source of variance was rooted in the biological rather than technical reproducibility. The technical reproducibility of the label-free method was very high at CV 10-13%, whereas the biological reproducibility (including the whole *N*-glycosite isolation process) was somewhat lower at CV below 25%. Therefore, protein abundance changes of 50% and more could be reliably assigned. These data, achieved with samples isolated via a complex sample preparation method are consistent with data

4 - Label-free quantitative cell surface proteomics

obtained with much simpler sample preparation protocols[34], indicating that the CSC method has a level of reproducibility that is compatible with label-free quantification. Several aspects of the data also suggest that the method chosen is sensitive. First, we were able to quantify a higher number of N-glycosites and proteins than with the isotope labeling method. This was the result of the possibility of propagating MS1 features identified in one pattern or for that matter represented in the cell surface atlas over all the other patterns in the study[20]. Second, we were able to identify and quantify GPCR proteins that are known to be expressed in levels numbering in the upper hundreds to low thousands of copies per cell[33], and third, the method displayed a dynamic range exceeding three orders of magnitude. Furthermore, a higher number of peptides could be quantified using the label-free method. At least in part this excellent sensitivity and dynamic range could be due to reduced ion suppression effects that are the result of the reduced sample complexity.

We used the combination of label-free quantitative mass spectrometry with CSC to test the hypothesis that the perturbation of signaling systems in the cell could be detected by quantitative changes in the cell surface proteome. Importantly, the method does not necessarily show differences in protein abundance but rather differences in the amount of the respective glycopeptides between samples which could arise from changes in the protein concentration or changes in glycosylation site occupancy. Perturbation of cultured *D. melanogaster* cells with different well-characterized chemicals known to change important intracellular signaling systems indeed affected the cell surface glyco-proteome in a specific manner. With one for the perturbations, the stimulation of Kc167 cells with insulin, we further attempted to distinguish different fates of proteins that showed quantitative changes on the cell surface. This was accomplished by comparing the quantitative pattern of cell surface proteins via CSC following insulin stimulation with the pattern of the same glycoproteins in the whole cell membrane using N-glycosite capturing. For InR we observed internalization but not significant degradation, a pattern that is in agreement with the findings observed by Knutson et al.[45] who used a heavy-isotope density-shift technique. Furthermore, we observed additional cell surface glycoproteins exhibiting similar behavior as InR and proteins showing different fates. Notable is the protein roundabout which showed a pattern opposite to InR suggesting that it might undergo exocytosis. By combining whole cell membrane and cell surface N-glycosite measurement we could therefore monitor biologically relevant quantitative changes and at least in part determine the underlying rationale for different patters such as internalization without degradation, protein degradation or intracellular redistribution.

In conclusion, we could assign a specific fingerprint indicating a cells origin, function and physical state using our proteomics and informatics pipeline. Cell surface proteins are carrying out various important functions and are therefore important targets in many pharmacological studies. The findings in this study indicate that the cell surface proteome mirrors changes occurring within the cell. Since at least some of the cell surface glycoproteins are also secreted, shed or otherwise released by the cell the systematic analysis of this important subproteome therefore opens the possibility of detecting molecular signatures in body fluids indicating the state of a cell or tissue. These results presented here are therefore of interest for the wide field of biomarker discovery where large research efforts are currently being invested.

4.7 References

1. Schiess, R. et al. Analysis of cell surface proteome changes via label-free, quantitative mass spectrometry. *Mol Cell Proteomics* **8**, 624-38 (2009).
2. Aebersold, R.H. & Mann, M. Mass spectrometry-based proteomics. *Nature* **422**, 198-207 (2003).
3. de Godoy, L.M. et al. Status of complete proteome analysis by mass spectrometry: SILAC labeled yeast as a model system. *Genome Biol* **7**, R50 (2006).
4. Schmidt, A. et al. An integrated, directed mass spectrometric approach for in-depth characterization of complex peptide mixtures. *Mol Cell Proteomics* (2008).
5. Mueller, L.N., Brusniak, M.Y., Mani, D.R. & Aebersold, R.H. An Assessment of Software Solutions for the Analysis of Mass Spectrometry Based Quantitative Proteomics Data. *J Proteome Res* **7**, 51-61 (2008).
6. Zhang, H. et al. High throughput quantitative analysis of serum proteins using glycopeptide capture and liquid chromatography mass spectrometry. *Mol Cell Proteomics* **4**, 144-55 (2005).
7. Gygi, S.P. et al. Quantitative analysis of complex protein mixtures using isotope-coded affinity tags. *Nat Biotechnol* **17**, 994-9 (1999).
8. Bodenmiller, B., Mueller, L.N., Mueller, M., Domon, B. & Aebersold, R.H. Reproducible isolation of distinct, overlapping segments of the phosphoproteome. *Nat Methods* **4**, 231-7 (2007).
9. Zhang, H., Li, X.J., Martin, D.B. & Aebersold, R.H. Identification and quantification of N-linked glycoproteins using hydrazide chemistry, stable isotope labeling and mass spectrometry. *Nat Biotechnol* **21**, 660-6 (2003).
10. McDonald, L., Robertson, D.H., Hurst, J.L. & Beynon, R.J. Positional proteomics: selective recovery and analysis of N-terminal proteolytic peptides. *Nat Methods* **2**, 955-7 (2005).
11. Marelli, M., Nesvizhskii, A.I. & Aitchison, J.D. Identifying bona fide components of an organelle by isotope-coded labeling of subcellular fractions : an example in peroxisomes. *Methods Mol Biol* **432**, 357-71 (2008).
12. Kislinger, T. et al. Global survey of organ and organelle protein expression in mouse: combined proteomic and transcriptomic profiling. *Cell* **125**, 173-86 (2006).
13. Zola, H. et al. CD molecules 2005: human cell differentiation molecules. *Blood* **106**, 3123-6 (2005).
14. Brunner, E. et al. A high-quality catalog of the Drosophila melanogaster proteome. *Nat Biotechnol* **25**, 576-83 (2007).
15. Bodenmiller, B. et al. PhosphoPep--a phosphoproteome resource for systems biology research in Drosophila Kc167 cells. *Mol Syst Biol* **3**, 139 (2007).
16. Rinner, O. et al. An integrated mass spectrometric and computational framework for the analysis of protein interaction networks. *Nat Biotechnol* **25**, 345-52 (2007).
17. Gygi, S.P., Corthals, G.L., Zhang, Y., Rochon, Y. & Aebersold, R.H. Evaluation of two-dimensional gel electrophoresis-based proteome analysis technology. *Proc Natl Acad Sci U S A* **97**, 9390-5 (2000).
18. Wollscheid, B. et al. Mass-spectrometric identification and relative quantification of N-linked cell surface glycoproteins. *Nat Biotechnol* **27**, 378-86 (2009).
19. Gahmberg, C.G. & Tolvanen, M. Why mammalian cell surface proteins are glycoproteins. *Trends Biochem Sci* **21**, 308-11 (1996).
20. Mueller, L.N. et al. SuperHirn - a novel tool for high resolution LC-MS-based peptide/protein profiling. *Proteomics* **7**, 3470-80 (2007).
21. Arsenis, G., Hayes, G.R. & Livingston, J.N. Insulin receptor cycling and insulin action in the rat adipocyte. *J Biol Chem* **260**, 2202-7 (1985).
22. Radimerski, T. et al. Identification of insulin-induced sites of ribosomal protein S6 phosphorylation in Drosophila melanogaster. *Biochemistry* **39**, 5766-74 (2000).
23. Schmidt, A., Kellermann, J. & Lottspeich, F. A novel strategy for quantitative proteomics using isotope-coded protein labels. *Proteomics* **5**, 4-15 (2005).

4 - Label-free quantitative cell surface proteomics

24. Pedrioli, P.G. et al. A common open representation of mass spectrometry data and its application to proteomics research. *Nat Biotechnol* **22**, 1459-66 (2004).
25. Eng, J.K., McCormack, A.L. & Yates, J.R. An approach to correlate tandem mass spectral data of peptides with amino acid sequences in a protein database. *J Am Soc Mass Spectrom* **5**, 976-89 (1994).
26. Keller, A., Eng, J.K., Zhang, N., Li, X.J. & Aebersold, R.H. A uniform proteomics MS/MS analysis platform utilizing open XML file formats. *Mol Syst Biol* **1**, 2005.0017 (2005).
27. Keller, A., Nesvizhskii, A.I., Kolker, E. & Aebersold, R.H. Empirical statistical model to estimate the accuracy of peptide identifications made by MS/MS and database search. *Anal Chem* **74**, 5383-92 (2002).
28. Nesvizhskii, A.I., Keller, A., Kolker, E. & Aebersold, R.H. A statistical model for identifying proteins by tandem mass spectrometry. *Anal Chem* **75**, 4646-58 (2003).
29. Han, D.K., Eng, J.K., Zhou, H. & Aebersold, R.H. Quantitative profiling of differentiation-induced microsomal proteins using isotope-coded affinity tags and mass spectrometry. *Nat Biotechnol* **19**, 946-51 (2001).
30. Hirokawa, T., Boon-Chieng, S. & Mitaku, S. SOSUI: classification and secondary structure prediction system for membrane proteins. *Bioinformatics* **14**, 378-9 (1998).
31. Sonnhammer, E.L., Von Heijne, G. & Krogh, A. A hidden Markov model for predicting transmembrane helices in protein sequences. *Proc Int Conf Intell Syst Mol Biol* **6**, 175-82 (1998).
32. Al-Shahrour, F., Minguez, P., Vaquerizas, J.M., Conde, L. & Dopazo, J. BABELOMICS: a suite of web tools for functional annotation and analysis of groups of genes in high-throughput experiments. *Nucleic Acids Res* **33**, W460-4 (2005).
33. Stanasila, L., Pattus, F. & Massotte, D. Heterologous expression of G-protein-coupled receptors: human opioid receptors under scrutiny. *Biochimie* **80**, 563-71 (1998).
34. Wang, G., Wu, W.W., Zeng, W., Chou, C.L. & Shen, R.F. Label-free protein quantification using LC-coupled ion trap or FT mass spectrometry: Reproducibility, linearity, and application with complex proteomes. *J Proteome Res* **5**, 1214-23 (2006).
35. Chen, W., White, M.A. & Cobb, M.H. Stimulus-specific requirements for MAP3 kinases in activating the JNK pathway. *J Biol Chem* **277**, 49105-10 (2002).
36. Botella, J.A. et al. The Drosophila cell shape regulator c-Jun N-terminal kinase also functions as a stress-activated protein kinase. *Insect Biochem Mol Biol* **31**, 839-47 (2001).
37. Standaert, M.L. & Pollet, R.J. Equilibrium model for insulin-induced receptor down-regulation. Regulation of insulin receptors in differentiated BC3H-1 myocytes. *J Biol Chem* **259**, 2346-54 (1984).
38. Radimerski, T. et al. dS6K-regulated cell growth is dPKB/dPI(3)K-independent, but requires dPDK1. *Nat Cell Biol* **4**, 251-5 (2002).
39. Kolodziej, P.A. et al. frazzled encodes a Drosophila member of the DCC immunoglobulin subfamily and is required for CNS and motor axon guidance. *Cell* **87**, 197-204 (1996).
40. Burgess, J.W. et al. Decrease in beta-subunit phosphotyrosine correlates with internalization and activation of the endosomal insulin receptor kinase. *J Biol Chem* **267**, 10077-86 (1992).
41. Authier, F., Rachubinski, R.A., Posner, B.I. & Bergeron, J.J. Endosomal proteolysis of insulin by an acidic thiol metalloprotease unrelated to insulin degrading enzyme. *J Biol Chem* **269**, 3010-6 (1994).
42. Doherty, J.J., Kay, D.G., Lai, W.H., Posner, B.I. & Bergeron, J.J. Selective degradation of insulin within rat liver endosomes. *J Cell Biol* **110**, 35-42 (1990).
43. Tomiya, N., Narang, S., Lee, Y.C. & Betenbaugh, M.J. Comparing N-glycan processing in mammalian cell lines and native and engineered lepidopteran insect cell lines. *Glycoconj J* **21**, 343-60 (2004).
44. Medzihradszky, K.F. Characterization of site-specific N-glycosylation. *Methods Mol Biol* **446**, 293-316 (2008).
45. Knutson, V.P., Ronnett, G.V. & Lane, M.D. Control of insulin receptor level in 3T3 cells: effect of insulin-induced down-regulation and dexamethasone-induced up-regulation on rate of receptor inactivation. *Proc Natl Acad Sci USA* **79**, 2822-6 (1982).

5 Discovery and validation of protein biomarkers for prostate cancer diagnosis

5.1 Authorship

Here I applied the concepts and methods discussed in the previous chapters to discover new biomarkers for the diagnosis of prostate cancer. This project was an integrated collaborative effort including many different specialists. Together with Igor Cima who carried out the cell biology based experiments, I was the main contributor to this work and did the proteomics analysis. Reto Ossola helped me with the automated glycocapturing and Vinzenz Lange supported me with the targeted proteomics analysis. Importantly, the project was assisted by a strong clinical alliance of medical doctors, Silke Gillessen, Arnoud Templeton, Martin Kälin, and Peter Wild, which provided conclusive clinical knowledge. Ruedi Aebersold (IMSB) and Wilhelm Krek (Institute of Cell Biology) together with Thomas Cerny (Kantonsspital St. Gallen) and Holger Moch (University Hospital Zurich) supported this joint effort with excellent scientific advice.

5.2 Summary

The availability of protein biomarkers for the detection of early-stage cancer will have profound impact on human health, especially for tumors with silent progression such as prostate cancer. Blood is thought to pick up molecular cues or biomarkers as it circulates through the various tissues, collectively reflecting molecular processes active in those different tissues. To increase the proteomic detection sensitivity, we have developed a method for the selective analysis of N-glycosites from tissue and serum. The analysis of glycoproteins is ideally suited for the detection of such signatures because they are preferentially released from tissue and deposited in the bloodstream where they can be detected in a non-invasive fashion. In our study we initially used the *Pten* conditional knock-out (cKO) mouse model for prostate cancer progression. This model in which the different stages of the disease can be deliberately and reproductively induced and followed, allowed us to simulate with very high fidelity the early steps of the human disease. Under the assumption that proteins of interest are enriched in the tissue, we performed label-free comparative proteomics of $Pten^{-/-}$ and control tissue at different time points. Interesting candidates were then monitored in the corresponding mice sera by targeted mass spectrometry using Selected Reaction Monitoring (SRM) at high sensitivity and selectivity. Finally, we showed that a protein signature consisting of Protein-lysine 6-oxidase (LOX), Vitronectin (VTN) and Asporin (ASPN) in combination with PSA predicted localized prostate cancer more precisely than current tests. These results clearly illustrates that the use of mouse models in combination with in-depth quantitative MS analysis of glycoproteins and targeted MS thereof provides a useful strategy to identify candidate markers applicable to human cancer.

5.3 Introduction

Prostate cancer is the most commonly diagnosed cancer in men. Moreover, it is the second leading cause of cancer deaths in men[1]. Its development proceeds through a series of defined steps, including prostatic intraepithelial neoplasia (PIN), invasive cancer and hormone-dependent or -independent metastasis. The treatment of cancers confined to the prostate gland typically involves radical prostatectomy, external beam radiotherapy or brachytherapy. While many patients with localized disease require no additional treatment, a subgroup will relapse and develop distant metastatic disease. Relapsed patients or patients who present with metastatic disease are treated by withdrawal of androgenic hormones. While the majority of patients will respond to androgen ablation, responses eventually give way to progressive, hormone-refractory prostate cancer.

Despite advances over the past decade, treatment options for advanced prostate cancer are inadequate, the side effects of treatment are significant and often unacceptable, and troubling questions remain about the efficacy of early detection for the disease. The limited knowledge about the causes of prostate cancer, how it may be detected and prevented at early stage, and how to treat it successfully demand new integrated approaches that span basic science, technology development and clinical research in order to develop informative biomarkers and effective therapies for this disease.

Prostate-specific antigen (PSA) is one of the few molecular markers routinely used for detection, risk stratification and monitoring of prostate cancer. PSA is specific for prostate but not to prostate cancer. Benign prostate diseases such as benign prostatic hyperplasia (BPH) often cause increases in serum PSA leading to a substantial "overdiagnosis" of prostate cancer[2]. Due to its high false-positive prediction, three out of four patients undergo unnecessary biopsy.

Among the most frequent genetic alterations in human prostate cancer are *PTEN* tumor suppressor gene mutations. The major function of PTEN relies on its phosphatase activity toward PIP3 (phosphatidyl inositol 3,4,5,-triphosphate) and, consequently, antagonism of the PI3K (phosphatidylinositol 3-kinase) signaling pathway, which is normally activated by growth factors including insulin-like growth factor (IGF) 1. Loss of PTEN function results in accumulation of PIP3 and the activation of downstream effectors such as the protein kinase AKT/PKB, which phosphorylates key effector proteins leading to increased cell metabolism, cell growth, proliferation, survival and invasiveness. Among the effector

5 – Discovery and validation of protein biomarkers for prostate cancer diagnosis 95

proteins inhibited by AKT/PKB is TSC2. TSC2 contributes to the negative regulation of the mTOR (mammalian target of rapamycin) pathway, that regulates protein translation, transcription, autophagy and cell growth as a function of nutrients and energy status. Accordingly, inactivation of PTEN results in an AKT/PKB-dependent activation of mTOR and a resulting deregulation of cell growth and proliferation. In this pathway, furthest along in development among the potentially targeted therapeutics in prostate cancer are inhibitors of mTOR such as CCI-779, RAD001 and AP23573, all of which are derivatives of rapamycin[3].

Consistent with the view that Pten inactivation has particular relevance to prostate cancer initiation and progression are results derived from murine models of prostate cancers by deleting the *Pten* tumor suppressor gene specifically in the prostatic epithelium. This Pten-dependent prostate cancer model recapitulates many features of the disease progression seen in humans with defined kinetics[4]. Similar to human cancer, $Pten^{-/-}$ murine prostate cancers regress in response to androgen ablation therapy but subsequently relapse and proliferate in the absence of androgens. Taken together, these lines of evidence suggest that alterations of Pten or components of the pathway it operates in play a causal role in human prostate carcinogenesis and that the Pten-dependent prostate cancer mouse model represents a suitable inroad to cancer therapeutics and novel biomarkers in human prostate cancer. Here we put a major emphasis on the investigation of the impaired Pten signaling pathway in prostate cancer.

The search for novel potential biomarkers for the diagnosis of localized prostate cancer was carried out using extensive quantitative MS-based proteomic analysis strategy to tissues that were sampled from wildtype (wt) and prostate specific *Pten* conditional knock-out (cKO) mice. Under the assumption that proteins of interest are enriched in the tissue, our strategy was to use comparative proteomics of affected and control tissue. To increase the detection sensitivity of tissue-specific protein signatures in plasma, we used a method for the selective analysis of *N*-glycopeptides from tissue and plasma itself. The analysis of glycoproteins is ideally suited for the detection of such signatures because they are likely to be released from tissue and deposited in the bloodstream where they can be detected. Interesting candidates were then monitored by targeted mass spectrometry in serum at high sensitivity and selectivity. With this approach, we sought to explore the merits of the genetically defined *Pten* cKO model of prostate cancer to determine whether our proteomics technology allows identification of protein changes associated with tumor progression and whether such changes are relevant to human prostate cancer.

The human homologues of the protein marker candidates obtained from the mouse study were finally measured in the sera of patients with BPH and localized prostate cancer (locCaP). A protein signature consisting of Protein-lysine 6-oxidase (LOX), Vitronectin (VTN) and Asporin (ASPN) in combination with PSA was found to predict locCaP more precisely than current tests. Herewith, we could clearly demonstrate that the results obtained from the study using a mouse models in combination with in-depth quantitative MS analysis of glycoproteins and targeted MS thereof were valid for markers applicable to human cancer.

5.4 Experimental procedures

Chemicals. Porcine trypsin, modified, sequencing grade, was purchased from Promega (Madison, WI, USA). Tris(2-carboxyethyl)phosphine (TCEP), iodoacetamide and α-cyano-4-hydroxycinnamic acid were purchased from Fluka (Buchs, Switzerland). HPLC-grade water and acetonitrile were purchased from Riedel-de Haën (Seelze, Germany), sodium periodate (Perbio, Switzerland), RapiGest (Waters), PNGase F (NEB), Affi-Prep Hz Hydrazide (BioRad).

Generation of prostate-specific *Pten* exon 5 deletion $Pten^{lox/lox};Cre^+$ mice. To generate $Pten^{lox/lox};Cre^+$ mice, *ARR2Probasin-Cre* transgenic line, $PB\text{-}Cre4^5$ on *C57BL/6xDBA2* background were crossed to $Pten^{lox/lox}$ mice on a *129/Balb/c* background. The males offspring with $Pten^{lox/+};Cre^+$ genotype were then crossed to $Pten^{lox/lox}$ females. Only F2 generation of male offspring was used in this study.

Tissue and blood extraction procedure from mice. Mice were anesthetized and blood was extracted by pinning the left heart ventricle. Mice were subsequently heart-perfused. This allowed for the complete removal of blood from the prostate tissue. Tissue samples were then dissected and pure prostate tissue was readily snap frozen and pulverized by using a mortar and pestle in the presence of liquid nitrogen. Serum was extracted from the blood after complete clotting on ice and stored at -80°C until use.

Glycoprotein enrichment from tissue and serum. Murine prostate tissue was subjected to glycoprotein extraction using 50% trifluorethanol (TFE) for 2 hours at 60°C. Proteins were solubilized using RapiGest and proteolyzed with trypsin. Solid phase extraction of glycopeptides (SPEG) was performed as follows: Glycan moieties of glycopeptides were oxidized and coupled to hydrazide beads. Non-glycopeptides and tissue debris were washed away. *N*-linked glycopeptides were then released via *N*-Glycosidase F (PNGase F) and the recovered peptides analyzed by LC-MS/MS.

Glycoproteins were enriched from serum using the protocol published by H. Zhang et al.[6]. Glycoproteins were oxidized by adding sodium periodate. After removal of sodium periodate, the sample was conjugated to the hydrazide resin. Nonglycoproteins were then removed by washing the resin. Trypsin was added and the glycoproteins digested directly on the solid-phase resin. The trypsin released peptides were removed by washing the resin. *N*-linked glycopeptides were then released via PNGase F

5 – Discovery and Validation of protein biomarkers for prostate cancer diagnosis

and the recovered peptides analyzed by LC-MS/MS. Importantly, the protocol was implemented into a robotic platform (MultiPROBE II PLUS HT EX from Perkin Elmer) in order to get high reproducibility.

Mass spectrometry analysis. Samples were analyzed on a hybrid LTQ-FT mass spectrometer (Thermo Electron, San Jose, CA) equipped with a nanoelectrospray ion source. Chromatographic separation of peptides was performed on an Agilent 1100 micro HPLC system (Waldbronn, Germany), equipped with a 15 cm fused silica emitter, 150 µm inner diameter, packed with a Magic C18 AQ 5 µm resin (Michrom BioResources, Auburn, CA, USA). Peptides were loaded on the column from a cooled (4°C) Agilent autosampler and separated with a linear gradient of acetonitrile/water, containing 0.1% formic acid, at a flow rate of 1.2 µl/min. A linear gradient from 2 to 40% acetonitrile in 60 min which was optimized for the number of peptide features detected was used. The MS instrument was operated to maximize the quality of LC-MS feature maps as opposed to maximizing the number of identifications. Therefore, for each peptide sample a standard data-dependent acquisition (DDA) on the three most intense ions per MS-scan was performed. Three MS/MS spectra were acquired in the linear ion trap per FT-MS scan, the latter acquired at 100'000 FWHM (at 350 m/z) nominal resolution, resulting in an overall cycle time of approximately 1 second. Charge state screening was employed, allowing fragmentation of doubly and higher charged ions, and rejecting ions of single and unknown charge state. A threshold of 200 ion counts was set to trigger an MS/MS attempt.

Protein identification. The raw data acquired by the LTQ-FT (software: Xcalibur 2.0 SR1) was converted to mzXML using ReAdW 3.5.1[7] applying default parameters. MS/MS scans were then exported as .dta files without further processing using the program mzXML2Other[7]. MS/MS spectra were searched against the International Protein Index (IPI) murine protein database (version 3.26) using SEQUEST v.27[8]. The SEQUEST database search criteria included static modifications of 57.02146 Da for cysteines (for the alkylation with iodoacetamide) and variable modficiations of 15.99491 Da for methionines (for oxidation), and of 0.98406 Da for potential formerly N-glycosylated asparagines (which are converted to aspartic acid by PNGase F release), respectively. The following additional search constraints were applied: monoisotopic parent and fragment masses, precursor-ion mass tolerance: 0.05 Da, fragment-ion mass tolerance 0.5 Da, at least 1 tryptic terminus, 1 missed cleavage. The identified peptides were processed and analyzed through the mass spectrometry Trans-Proteomic Pipeline 3.5 (TPP)[9]. In the TPP, the database search results were validated using the PeptideProphet software[10], which uses various SEQUEST scores (XCorr, ΔCn, Sp) to calculate a probability score for each identified peptide by linear discriminant analysis. N-glycosylation motif information and accurate mass binning were used in PeptideProphet. The peptides were then assigned for protein identification using the ProteinProphet software[11]. ProteinProphet allowed filtering of large-scale data sets with assessment of predictable sensitivity and false positive identification error rates. In this study, we used a PeptideProphet probability score ≥ 0.9, and a ProteinProphet probability score ≥ 0.9. This resulted in an overall false positive error rate below 1% as determined by ProteinProphet[11].

Label-free quantification of peptide and protein ratios. Data from LC-MS runs were converted from raw to the mzXML data format[7] and processed by the software tool SuperHirn as described before[12]. JRatio was used for the calculation and visual assessment of peptide and protein ratios[13]. A normal distribution was used to describe the calculated protein ratios and t-student test statistics was applied to assess the significance of a protein fold change. Proteins with a P-Value ≤ 0.15 were considered to be significantly regulated.

In order to verify the results obtained by SuperHirn and JRatio, we performed spectral counting analysis. For every LC-MS/MS run, the ratio between total peptides for the protein to be quantified and the total peptides detected in the run was calculated. The average ratio from all the LC-MS/MS runs from all mice analyzed was calculated. The averaged ratio from $Pten^{-/-}$ mice was subtracted from the averaged ratio from $Pten^{+/+}$ mice. A positive difference for the ratio was considered as up-regulation for the selected protein. A one-tailed student's T test with unequal variances was applied to calculate the level of significance of the detected differences. A non-stringent P-value ≤ 0.15 was considered statistically significant.

mRNA analysis of prostatic mouse tissue. Prostate tissue was dissected from hearth-perfused mice, and pure prostatic tissue was subjected to total RNA extraction using the RNeasy minikit (QIAGEN) following the manufacturer instructions. 2 μg of total RNA was subjected to reverse transcription using the Ready-To-Go You-Prime First-Strand beads (GE Healthcare). cDNA was used to amplify specific targets by real-time PCR using SYBR green I master mix (Roche), the 480 light cycler (Roche) and following primer pairs for RT-PCR of *Thormbospondin (Thbs1)* cDNA:
Forward Primer: GGGGAGATAACGGTGTGTTTG
Reverse Primer: CGGGGATCAGGTTGGCATT

Immunofluorescence on cryosections. The upper genitourinary tract was dissected from wt and Pten cKO mice and readily frozen in OCT medium and stored at -80°C until use. 7 μm sections were fixed for 8 min in 4% PFA, 1% sucrose. To bloc unspecific binding of antibodies, the sections were blocked 30 min using a PBS solution at pH 7.4 containing 10% goat serum and 0.1% Triton-X-100. The primary antibody was incubated overnight at 4°C in blocking buffer. Fluorescently labeled secondary antibodies were used to detect the primary antibody bound to the antigen. Images were acquired using an Axioplan 2

5 – Discovery and validation of protein biomarkers for prostate cancer diagnosis 99

imaging system (Zeiss). The following antibodies were used: anti-CD44 (rat monoclonal: clone IM-7, eBioscience) and anti-Lamp-2 (rat monoclonal: clone GL2A7, DSHB).

Tissue microarray analysis. The TMA slide was obtained from the H. Moch (Department of Surgical Pathology, University Hospital Zurich) and stained with an anti-Periostin antibody (rabbit polyclonal from Biovendor). The TMA was analyzed with the Ventana Benchmark automated staining system (Ventana Medical Systems, Tucson, AZ) using Ventana reagents for the entire procedure[14].

Handling and preparation of human sera. All patients had to sign an informed consent. 8 ml blood were drawn and collected in a serum seperator tube containing clot activator and gel (Becton Dickinson, Allschwil, Switzerland). Tubes were inverted 8 times and centrifuged within 4 h of collection at 4°C for 10 min at 1428 rcf. The serum was divided in 5 aliquots 500 µl each and stored at -60°C or lower until use.

Targeted mass spectrometry analysis using SRM. We used the absolute quantification of proteins strategy (termed AQUA) introduced by Gerber et al.[15]. As internal standards we used at least one heavy labeled form of an N-glycosite per protein from Sigma-Aldrich, called AQUA peptide. In the beginning, we used these AQUA peptides to optimize the SRM-transitions specific for each N-glycosite that were formerly generated *in silico* using TIQAM software[16]. For each AQUA-peptide precursor we calculated the transitions with precursor charges 2+ and 3+ and the four smallest y-ions with m/z > precursor m/z + 30. Collision energies were calculated according to the formulas: CE = 0.044 * m/z + 5.5 (2+) and CE = 0.051 * m/z + 0.5 (3+). Then, we optimized 100 transitions per run on a pool of all six serum samples varying the dwell-time and the collision energy. Results were imported into TIQAM and the three transitions with the best signal/noise ratio were selected for quantitative analysis. For quantitative analysis we spiked heavy peptides as internal standard to each serum sample. For each AQUA-peptide transition we calculated the corresponding transition of the endogenouse peptide. This resulted in six transitions per peptide. By restricting the acquisition of each transition to a 2-3 minute window around its elution time, the time scheduling feature of the acquisition software enabled the analysis of all transitions in a single run per sample without compromising on sensitivity.

SRM analyses were performed on a hybrid triple quadrupole/linear ion trap mass spectrometer 4000 Q TRAP operated with a beta release of Analyst 1.4.2 supporting scheduled experiments (Applied Biosystems/MDS Sciex). The instrument was coupled to a Tempo Nano LC system (Applied Biosystems/MDS Sciex) for peptide separation using a 30 min gradient from 5 to 30 % acetonitrile (0.1% formic acid) at 300 nl/min flow rate. A fused silica emitter of 75 µm inner diameter was packed in-house with 13 cm Reprosil-Pur 120 ODS-3.3 um (Dr. Maisch GmbH). Quantitative analyses in SRM mode were performed with Q1 and Q3 operated in unit resolution (0.7 m/z half maximum peak width).

For quantification peak height was determined with Multiquant software (Vers. 1.1.0.16, Applied Biosystems/MDS Sciex) after confirming for each peptide the co-elution of all transitions. Peptides with unfavorable elution profile (bad resolution) or interfering noise in the heavy or light transitions were excluded from further data analysis and from the transition table. No individual outlier data points were removed. Calculation of the ratio of (peak height light transition) / (peak height heavy transition) to correct for spray efficiency and ionization differences between runs was used for normalization and quantification of absolute protein concentrations.

ELISA. Human Thrombospondin-1 (TSP-1) was detected in serum by means of a competitive ELISA. Human serum was diluted 1:400 in 1% BSA and incubated over night with a monoclonal mouse anti-human TSP-1 antibody (clone HB8432, Lab Vision). The antibody-antigen complex was then transferred on a plate coated with recombinant TSP-1 (R&D Systems) for 2 h to detect the unbound anti-TSP-1 antibody fraction. Signals were detected by anti-mouse antibodies conjugated with horseradish peroxidase and a suitable substrate according to the manufacturer's protocol.

Statistical analysis. Statistical analyses were performed using the SYSTAT 12.0 and the SPSS 14.0 softwares. The panel of proteins discriminating best between BPH and locCaP patients was found using linear discriminant analysis and applying the automatic stepwise modeling provided by the SYSTAT software, as well as a forward logistic regression approach using the likelihood ratio test with the SPSS software. Quadratic discriminant analysis was used to calculated specificity and sensitivity. To avoid biased results due to over-fitting of the model, the leave-one-out cross validation method was used. Classification of patients was also determined using a multivariate logistic regression model (formula 1) with the variable z (formula 2) that represents the different protein markers, while $f(z)$ represents the probability of a particular outcome, given that set of protein markers.

$$f(z) = \frac{1}{1+e^{-z}} \quad (1)$$

$$z = \beta_0 + \beta_1 x_1 + \beta_2 x_2 + \beta_3 x_3 + \cdots + \beta_k x_k \quad (2)$$

5.5 Results

5.5.1 Pten-loss induced prostate cancer mouse model

We chose to study the role of *PTEN* deletion in human prostate cancer by using a mouse model for 5 major reasons. First, in contrast to human, confined breeding conditions and controlled environmental changes result in a homogenous genetic background and eliminate important sources of variation that make human-based biomarker discoveries very challenging. Second, controlled and standardized tissue and blood sampling to limit any further sample heterogeneity. Third, defined stages of tumor development as genetic alterations associated with human tumors can be engineered in mice as demonstrated in resulting in defined perturbations. Fourth, in contrast to *in vitro* assays, the *in vivo* system promises to elucidate a repertoire of protein changes that occur in tissue and blood. Fifth, *PTEN* deletion and/or mutations are found in up to 60% of primary prostate cancers[17] and even more pronounced in metastatic prostate tissue samples showing its high relevance to human prostate cancer[18, 19].

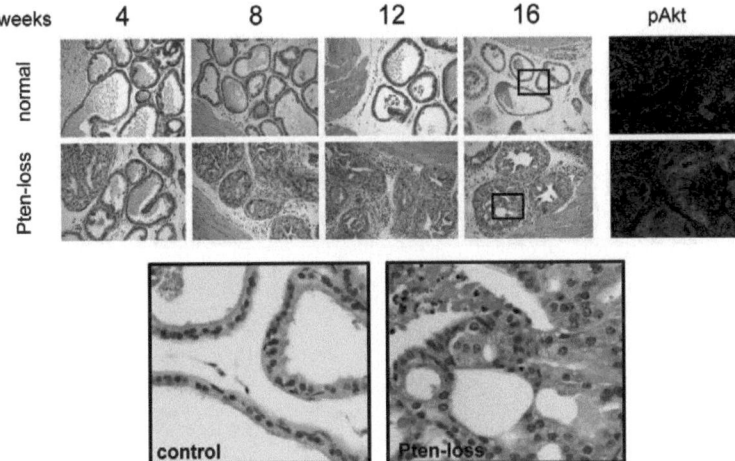

Figure 5.1 Comparison of pathological phenotype of 4- to 16-week-old *Pten$^{-/-}$* and *Pten$^{+/+}$* mice. *Pten* deletion in the murine prostate is achieved during puberty, at 6-8 weeks of age. The constitutive downstream activation of Akt (pAkt) shown in the upper right panel leads to an increased proliferation of the basal and luminal epithelial cell compartments. The cells fill up the luminal space and grow in a cribriform manner. Eventually, necrotic tissue can be seen (see zoom). The tumor however, does not become invasive, and its development can be compared to the early steps of prostate cancer progression, the so-called human high-grade prostatic intraepithelial neoplasia (HGPIN), a precursor of invasive prostate carcinoma. The cellular phenotype moreover,

closely resembles the classical human malignant prostate cancer cell, with enlarged cell size and nuclei, prominent nucleoli, organized in a cribriform manner.

The conditional deletion of *Pten* tumor suppressor was studied in a mouse model employing the *Cre/lox* system in order to control tissue-specific gene expression. Figure 5.1 illustrates the *Pten* deletion dependant development of PINs and localized prostate cancer in a $Pten^{-/-}$ compared to a $Pten^{+/+}$ mouse and thus the different early stages of the disease can be deliberately and reproductively induced and followed.

5.5.2 Proteomic analysis of mouse tissue and serum

We performed solid phase extraction of *N*-glycopeptides (SPEG) from the prostatic tissues and the corresponding sera of 3 $Pten^{+/+}$, 3 $Pten^{-/-}$ mice at 8 weeks of age and 3 $Pten^{+/+}$, 3 $Pten^{-/-}$ mice at 18 weeks of age. The *N*-glycosites from each sample were analyzed in duplicates on a LTQ-FTICR mass spectrometer. The proteomics-based glycoprotein enrichment technology in combination with high-throughput MS at a ProteinProphet[11] cutoff ≥ 0.9 resulted in the identification of 785 glycoproteins in total. 642 glycoproteins were detected in prostate tissue and 253 in serum. 110 proteins were detected in both the tissue as well as in the serum as illustrated in Figure 5.2. Figure 5.2 also shows the distribution of the glycoproteins in respect to their GO annotated cellular localization. More than 75% of the glycoproteins identified from tissue are predicted to be either secreted, to reside in the cell membrane, or to belong to compartments involved in the secretory pathway, respectively. In case of the serum the amount of glycoproteins to be specifically released or shed from the cell surface is even higher as it was expected. These results clearly illustrate that the glyco-proteome and in turn biomarker relevant proteins were enriched.

5 – Discovery and validation of protein biomarkers for prostate cancer diagnosis   103

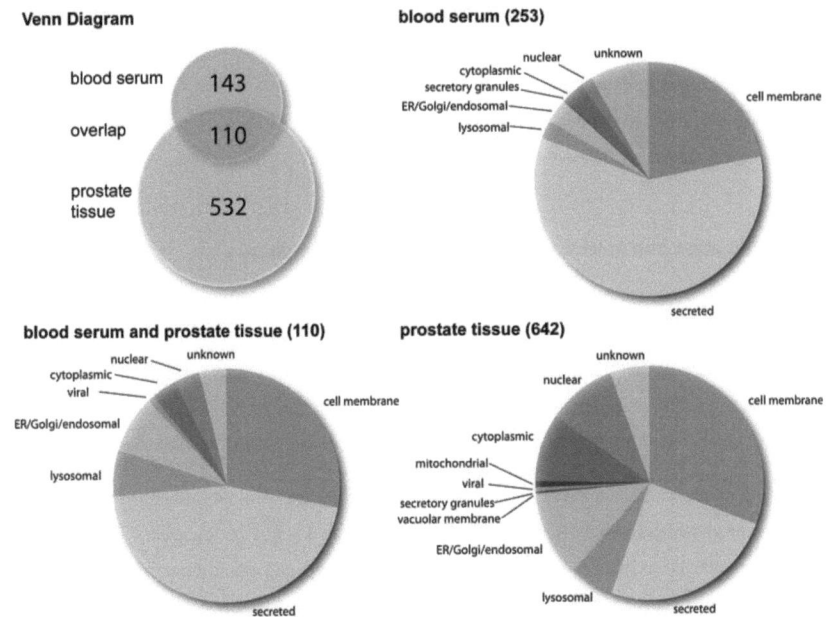

Figure 5.2 The Venn Diagram illustrates the number of glycoproteins identified from mouse blood serum and mouse prostate tissue including their overlap. The pie charts show the GO annotated cellular locations of glycoproteins identified blood serum, prostate tissue, or in both.

In order to find potential prostate cancer marker candidates, we performed label-free quantitative MS proteomics analysis of the glycoproteins identified before. Two different time points (8 and 18 weeks of age) were evaluated to get early as well as late cancer indicating protein signatures. Two approaches for label-free protein quantification were applied: First, glycoprotein abundance differences were calculated by comparing peptide elution ion trace profiles among the different samples using the SuperHirn software as described in chapter 4. In total, we were able to quantify 352 proteins (213 tissue/105 serum/ 34 both) by using this computational approach. Second, we also performed spectral counting[20, 21] to verify the elution profile comparison based results (see Supplementary Table S5.1). Potential candidates for prostate cancer diagnosis were selected primarily from the quantitative experiments where abundance ratios at either 8 or 18 weeks of age were observed. Thereby up- or down-regulated proteins in tumor samples were treated alike. We used a non-stringent P-value cutoff of ≤ 0.15 to avoid the loss of interesting candidates for later validation assays. In fact, all candidates will undergo further rigorous testing. Additional selection criteria for proteins supposed to be interesting candidates for further analysis included secreted proteins, proteins already detected in serum by conventional LC-MS/MS experiments, proteins being tissue specific to prostate according to large-scale analysis of human and mouse transcriptomes[22] represented in the GNF SymAtlas (http://symatlas.gnf.org/SymAtlas/) or proteins known to be biologically involved in cancer progression of any kind. On the basis of this evidence, we selected 164 proteins for further evaluation out of the 785 glycoproteins discovered (see Supplementary Table S5.1).

5.5.3 Verification and selection of promising marker candidates

Further verification of interesting proteins was performed using different techniques. Additional information from RT-PCR and immunhistochemistry (IHC) based experiments was used to add additional filter criteria for candidate selection in order to restrict the number of proteins of interest and focus further validation on promising marker candidates. This step was necessary because the number of proteins that can be validated by MS or antibody-based assays is still limited by time and money.

A first promising candidate selected for further investigation was Thrombospondin-1 (Tsp-1). Pten is known to control the expression of Tsp-1, a known negative regulator of angiogenesis[23]. Moreover, Tsp-1 is a well characterized p53 target gene[24]. Along with Pten-loss, we and others detected a concomitant p53 activation in the mouse prostate following Pten-loss, indicating a potential contribution of the p53 response axis in shaping the prostate glyco-proteome[25] (results not shown). MS analysis revealed exclusive expression of Tsp-1 in the tissue of $Pten^{-/-}$ mice. Two distinct N-glycosites, K.VVN*STTGPGEHLR and K.VSCPIMPCSN*ATVPDGECCPR were solely identified and quantified in the glycoprotein enriched samples from mice with Pten-loss at 8 and 18 weeks (Figure 5.3a). mRNA analysis of prostatic mouse tissue revealed a 6-fold up-regulation in cancerous tissue and was thus in agreement with the proteomic results Figure 5.3b.

5 – Discovery and Validation of protein biomarkers for prostate cancer diagnosis   105

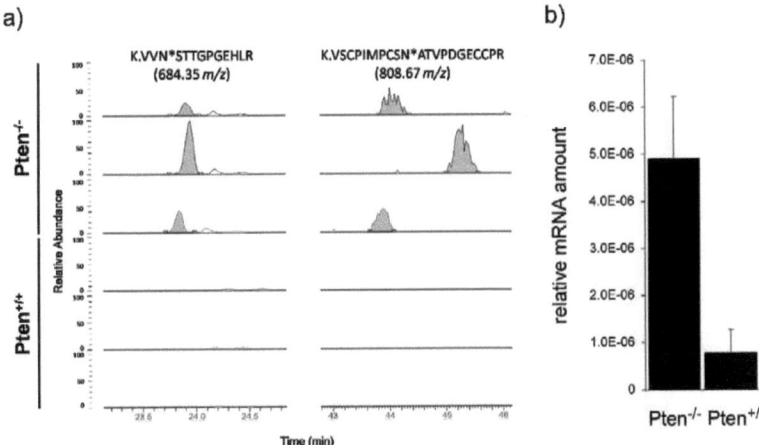

Figure 5.3 Thrombospondin-1 (Tsp-1) expression levels in prostate tissue at protein and mRNA level. a) Mass spectrometric elution profile of two peptide ions originating from two different N-glycosites of Tsp-1 originating from 3 $Pten^{-/-}$ and 3 $Pten^{+/+}$ at 8 weeks of age. b) mRNA expression levels of the corresponding mouse prostate tissue from tumors and controls.

Two other interesting candidates identified by quantitative MS analysis of mouse prostate tissue and serum, CD44 and Lysosomal-associated membrane protein 2 (CD107b), were further verified by immunofluorescence. CD44 is an adhesion molecule known to be involved in cell proliferation, migration and invasion[26]. MS analysis revealed its up-regulation on the protein level in $Pten^{-/-}$ tissue compared to $Pten^{+/+}$ mouse tissue. As shown in Figure 5.4, CD44 was aberrantly expressed in the tissue of $Pten^{-/-}$ mice indicating a high tumorigenic potential. CD107b is a glycoprotein that may play a role in tumor cell metastasis and was more than three times up-regulated in cancerous tissue of $Pten^{-/-}$ mice compared to control mice in the label-free MS experiments. Staining of CD107b in tissue revealed a very strong staining in the tissue of $Pten^{-/-}$ mice being consistent with the MS results. These two examples nicely illustrate the correlation between conventional IHC-based experiments and quantitative MS analysis.

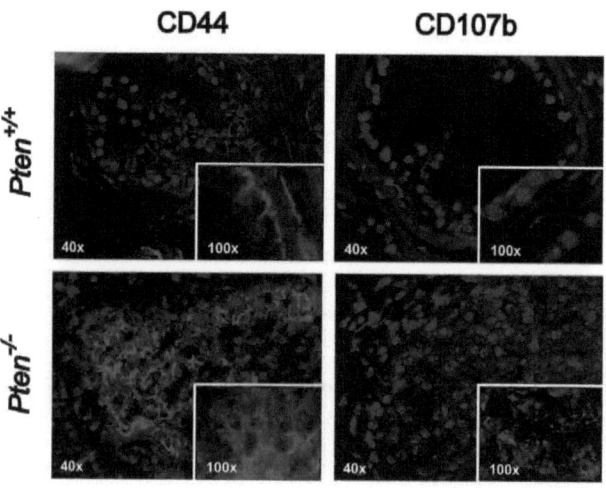

Figure 5.4 IHC staining of CD44 and CD107b in 8 weeks old $Pten^{+/+}$ and $Pten^{-/-}$ mouse tissue shows aberrant protein expression in mice with Pten-loss.

5.5.4 Verification of marker candidates by targeted MS in mouse serum

A major limiting step in biomarker discovery is the verification of markers discovered in high-throughput screens. Here we used targeted MS analysis using selected reaction monitoring (SRM). This novel approach allows the simultaneous detection and quantification of proteins comparable in sensitivity to classical immunodetection procedures (e.g. Enzyme-Linked ImmunoSorbent Assay, ELISA), but with the advantage of not requiring tedious optimization steps for each biomarker candidate and generation of new antibodies. However, for the routine measurements we still need to develop antibody-based assays but for the verification of promising marker candidates SRM is much faster. The SRM experiment is accomplished by specifying the parent mass of the compound for MS/MS fragmentation and then specifically monitoring for a single fragment ion. Thus, SRM delivers a unique fragment ion that can be monitored and quantified in the midst of a very complicated matrix. Stable isotope labeled peptides corresponding to the targeted N-glycosites were synthesized and used as internal standards for absolute quantification. We analyzed the sera of the corresponding 3 $Pten^{+/+}$, 3 $Pten^{-/-}$ mice at 8 weeks of age and 3 $Pten^{+/+}$, 3 $Pten^{-/-}$ mice at 18 weeks of age. The sera were enriched for N-glycosites as described before. In parallel, SRM assays for 60 different N-glycosites were established chosen from the list of 164

5 – Discovery and Validation of protein biomarkers for prostate cancer diagnosis

interesting candidates. 44 endogenous *N*-glycosites were detected and quantified in the glyco-enriched mouse serum samples and quantified (see Supplementary Table S5.2).

Besides Lysosome-associated membrane glycoprotein 1 (Lamp-1) that showed lower serum levels in $Pten^{-/-}$ mice, no significant changes (*P*-value < 0.05) among the proteins measured in 8 weeks old mice were found. This lack of changes was not surprising since we already knew from the pathological investigation of mouse tissue and the tissue proteomics-based protein quantification experiments that fewer changes occurred at an early state of disease compared to later stage. In contrast to the early disease stage, several proteins measured in 18 weeks old mice revealed significant differences (*P*-Value <0.05). As an example, Tsp-1, which was formerly found to be highly up-regulated in cancer bearing tissue, was 5-fold down-regulated (*P*-Value: 0.009) in the sera of $Pten^{-/-}$ mice. This opposite effect in serum compared with tissue was likely due to impaired Tsp-1 secretion that has been previously described to be decreased or absent in later prostate cancer stages[27]. Other interesting candidates were Cathepsin D (cancer/normal ratio: 2.3±0.8, *P*-Value: 0.010), Leukemia inhibitory factor receptor (2.6±0.8, 0.013), Receptor-type tyrosine-protein phosphatase kappa (2.2±0.6, 0.020), Glucosylceramidase (3.1±1.2, 0.023), Acid ceramidase (2.7±1.3, 0.023), Asporin (2.8±1.0, 0.026), Attractin (2.4±0.7, 0.027), Neural cell adhesion molecule 1 (2.5±1.0, 0.030), Extracellular matrix protein 1 (3.1±1.9, 0.033), Pancreatic lipase-related protein 1 (2.4±0.9, 0.037), Golgi phosphoprotein 2 (4.0±2.1, 0.048), and Low-density lipoprotein receptor-related protein 1 (2.2±0.9, 0.049). For the complete list of glycoprotein see Supplementary Table S5.2. Importantly, proteins being present at low blood serum concentrations of few ng/ml such as Tyrosine-protein phosphatase non-receptor type substrate 1 (2-4 ng/ml) were reliably detected. This performance is comparable to sensitivities achieved by ELISA and demonstrates the huge potential of the approach we applied.

5.5.5 ELISA and MS-based validation in human serum

As indicated earlier, the *Pten* cKO mouse model employed in this study allowed us to reliably recapitulate the early steps of human prostate cancer progression. The model enabled us to compare tissue and serum of cancer bearing and control mice in a highly reproducible fashion because mice can be sampled at defined stages of tumor development and under controlled breeding conditions. Here we wanted to demonstrate the strong concordance between mouse and human prostatic cancer in both tissue and circulating markers.

In order to validate our findings from the initial discovery phase in tissue and the various verification experiments performed in tissue using RT-PCR and IHC followed by SRM in mouse sera, we set out to quantify the proteins directly in human sera using again SRM. We tested two different serum sample cohorts. The first group consisted of serum samples obtained from 15 patients diagnosed with BPH. These were compared to a group of 16 patients with locCaP. The samples were enriched for N-glycosites by automated SPEG. We used the reciprocal BLAST analysis to find the potential human orthologues of the murine proteins as predicted by Ensembl (http://www.ensembl.org/). 122 isotopically heavy-labeled reference N-glycosites were obtained. 97 of these reference peptides could be successfully detected in serum. Finally, we were able to quantify 44 endogenous N-glycosites in patient sera. This allowed for the absolute quantification of 39 endogenous glycoproteins present in the human sera. Table 5.1 shows the proteins measured in human sera of BPH patients (n=15) and patients with locCaP (n=16). In order to compare our results with current ELISA technology, we analyzed 52 serum samples with both SRM and an ELISA for TSP-1. A significant (<0.00001) correlation (Pearson's r=0.732) between the results was thus obtained by the two different technologies.

Table 5.1 List of proteins analyzed by SRM in human sera of BPH (n=15) and locCaP (n=16) patients. Proteins highlighted in bold exhibited significant changes (P-value < 0.1) among the two patient groups.

Protein [a]	BPH		locCaP		P-Value
	Mean	Standard Deviation	Mean	Standard Deviation	
Type-1 angiotensin II receptor	171.1	161.0	111.9	70.2	0.190
A-kinase anchor protein 13	397.6	96.3	379.9	44.3	0.516
Membrane copper amine oxidase	**143.9**	**48.0**	**113.4**	**45.6**	**0.079**
Apolipoprotein B-100	**24057.3**	**16671.8**	**16472.9**	**5950.0**	**0.098**
Asporin	**58.6**	**16.3**	**72.8**	**17.7**	**0.028**
Attractin	1831.5	517.6	1608.2	436.8	0.203
Zinc-alpha-2-glycoprotein	11706.5	2926.4	9963.5	3748.3	0.162
Cell adhesion molecule 1	159.3	43.4	147.9	36.7	0.435
Carcinoembryonic antigen-related cell adhesion molecule 1	2528.2	1135.3	2681.7	1105.6	0.716
Complement factor H	89409.0	15691.6	92836.2	20995.0	0.613
Clusterin precursor	268851.1	51970.0	273820.2	66467.5	0.819
Ceruloplasmin	47719.0	10580.9	48821.4	11116.5	0.780
Carboxypeptidase M	280.9	139.7	865.3	1711.6	0.198
Cathepsin D	105.0	51.6	103.8	42.5	0.945
Extracellular matrix protein 1	641.1	202.4	714.4	213.2	0.335
Ephrin-A5	106.3	18.7	107.2	13.4	0.884
Coagulation factor V	455.3	192.7	451.8	191.6	0.960
GALNTL4	1205.8	2652.7	466.7	667.7	0.289
Golgi phosphoprotein 2	115.6	61.0	151.3	79.6	0.174
Eukaryotic peptide chain release factor GTP-binding subunit ERF3A	437.4	95.3	413.1	29.3	0.339
Hypoxia up-regulated protein 1	**28.7**	**6.6**	**36.9**	**13.8**	**0.045**
Mast/stem cell growth factor receptor	43.8	34.3	29.9	5.9	0.122
Prostate-specific antigen	124.6	37.6	115.7	45.6	0.559
Neural cell adhesion molecule L1	1940.1	2747.7	1377.6	1002.8	0.449
Galectin-3-binding protein	532.1	221.7	502.8	218.1	0.713
Protein-lysine 6-oxidase	**663.6**	**215.9**	**482.1**	**125.4**	**0.007**

(continued)

5 – Discovery and validation of protein biomarkers for prostate cancer diagnosis

Table 5.1 (continued)

Protein [a]	BPH		locCaP		P-Value
	Mean	Standard Deviation	Mean	Standard Deviation	
Prolow-density lipoprotein receptor-related protein 1	70.3	23.4	78.8	21.6	0.302
NALP2	497.6	251.5	547.3	215.4	0.558
Neural cell adhesion molecule 1	438.7	139.0	527.1	218.2	0.192
Olfactomedin-4	691.6	473.8	527.8	289.2	0.251
Plasma glutamate carboxypeptidase	525.5	169.9	578.4	205.4	0.443
Proactivator polypeptide	28122.1	7941.8	27074.8	2711.1	0.622
Semaphorin-4D	45.2	11.4	54.2	32.1	0.313
Transferrin	15090.3	4065.2	17296.4	4633.6	0.171
Transferrin receptor protein 1	9424.4	3573.0	8370.5	1329.1	0.279
Thrombospondin-1	4440.5	2126.1	5558.4	2049.8	0.154
Metalloproteinase inhibitor 1	818.1	273.1	871.2	230.0	0.562
TM9SF3 protein	272.1	108.3	348.8	112.5	**0.064**
Vitronectin	3301.6	1056.2	2382.6	750.1	**0.009**

[a] All protein concentrations in human serum reported in ng/ml.

Among the 39 proteins validated in human sera of BPH and locCaP patients, we looked for a panel of proteins exhibiting the highest possible discrimination power between the two groups of patients. The statistical analysis resulted in the identification of three proteins, Protein-lysine 6-oxidase (LOX), Vitronectin (VTN) and Asporin (ASPN), respectively. While LOX was a candidate chosen because of its known role in tumor suppression, VTN and ASPN were both detected in mouse serum and tissue and ASPN was additionally shown by SRM to be up-regulated in mouse serum of cancer bearing mice. All 3 proteins showed a significant differential expression (P-value < 0.05) in sera from human patients with locCaP compared to BPH as illustrated in Figure 5.5. LOX is an enzyme that initiates the cross-linking of collagens and Elastin via oxidative deamination. In addition to cross-linking extracellular matrix proteins, the encoded protein is supposed to have a dual role in both tumor suppression and metastasis promotion[28]. The second constituent of the protein panel is VTN, a cell adhesion and spreading factor found in serum and tissues through integrin binding. It is an inhibitor of the terminal cytolytic complement pathway and has been speculated to be involved in hemostasis and tumor malignancy[29]. ASPN belongs to the family of Leucine-Rich Repeat (LRR) proteins associated with the cartilage matrix and its gene has been shown to be up-regulated in lobular carcinomas, when compared with normal lobular cells in breast cancer[30].

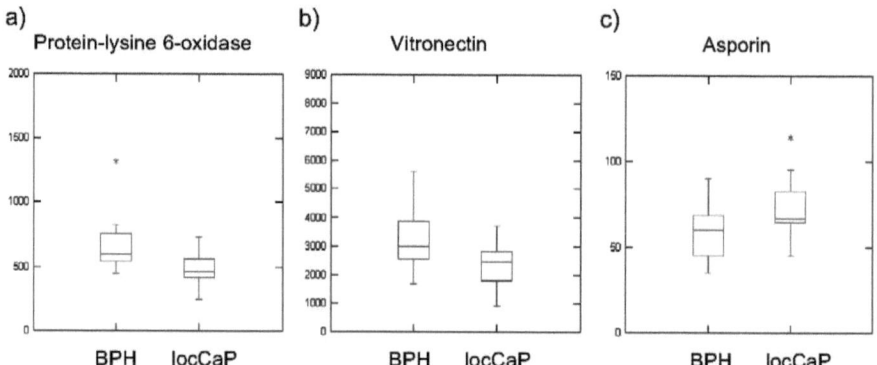

Figure 5.5 Box-plot analysis of differentially regulated proteins in BPH and locCaP. **a)** Protein-lysine 6-oxidase was down-regulated in locCaP patients (P-value 0.007). **b)** Vitronectin revealed lower protein expression in locCaP patients (P-value 0.009). **c)** Asporin was up-regulated in locCaP patients (P-value 0.028).

A multivariate model was created to distinguish between sera collected from the 31 patients with BPH (n=15) or locCaP (n=16). Using leave one-out cross-validation, the 3-biomarker signature had an accuracy of 84% (sens. 80%; spec. 81%), in comparison to PSA with an accuracy of 71% (sens. 90%; spec. 25%). By combining PSA with the 3-biomarker signature accuracy was further improved to 90% (sens. 93%; spec. 88%). We also calculated receiver operating characteristic curves for PSA levels in serum, the 3-biomarker signature as well as for the combination of PSA and the signature. The ability of the 3-biomarker signature alone was significant ($P<0.001$), with an area under the curve equal to 0.90 and 0.98 ($P<0.001$) for 3-biomarker signature in combination with PSA. The area under the curve for PSA was 0.84 ($P<0.001$) as shown in Figure 5.6.

5 – Discovery and validation of protein biomarkers for prostate cancer diagnosis

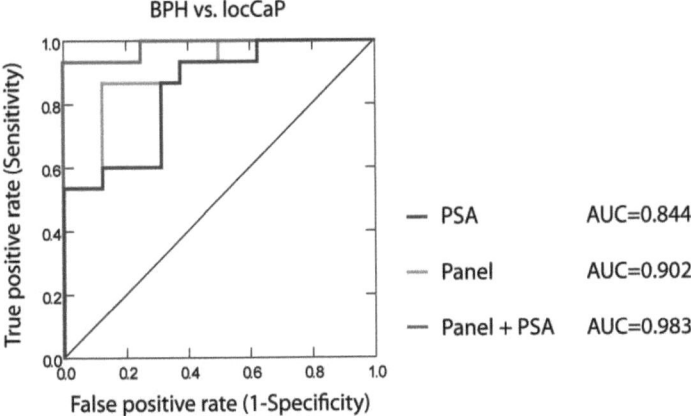

Figure 5.6 Receiver operating characteristic curve obtained from PSA (84% accuracy), the 3-biomarker panel consisting of ASN, VTN and LOX (90%) and the panel in combination with PSA (98%) in patients with BPH and locCaP.

These results clearly illustrate the superior performance of our new panel of proteins in respect to the diagnostic utility for prostate cancer by showing both higher sensitivity and specificity than PSA alone.

5.5.6 Periostin as a potential biomarker for prostate cancer staging

Differential diagnosis plays an increasingly important role as personalized medicine is on the rise. It is important to know if a patient has only BPH or prostate cancer because the way of disease treatment greatly differ. Periostin is particularly highly homologous to ßig-h3, which promotes cell adhesion and spreading of fibroblast, and has been reported to be frequently overexpressed in various types of human cancers[31]. We performed tissue microarray analysis (TMA) of Periostin in human to verify the unique identification by MS/MS of Periostin in sera from cancer bearing mice. Three different patient groups were compared in this experiment. The first patient group was diagnosed benign prostatic hyperplasia (BPH), while the patients in the second group had hormone sensitive prostate cancer (HSPC) and the ones in the third group hormone refractory prostate cancer (HRPC). In total 63 patients were tested (10 BPH, 30 HSPC, and 23 HRPC). The TMA analysis revealed an unambiguous overexpression of Periostin in patients diagnosed with prostate cancer. Figure 5.7a shows a section of the TMA slide analyzed. 9 out of 10 patients with BPH showed negative IHC staining for Periostin, while 87% of HSPC patients showed positive staining for Periostin and 83% of HRPC patients, respectively (Figure 5.7b). Again the MS results were confirmed.

Due to its low specificity, PSA serum screening has led to an increase of prostate needle biopsies in the last two decades. This in turn increased the rate of difficult diagnostic situations where immunohistochemical tests are necessary. Histological diagnosis of prostate cancer mainly rests on the conventional parameters of morphological architecture and cytology. However, cancer diagnosis can be problematic in some cases. Additional markers of prostate cancer are desirable[32]. The data presented here suggest Periostin as an additional ancillary positive marker for tissue-based diagnosis of prostate cancer.

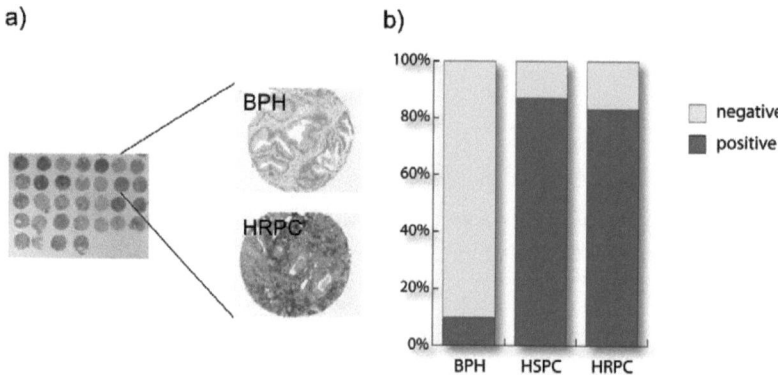

Figure 5.7 Periostin expression in prostate tissue at protein level. a) Section of a tissue microarray of 57 patients including 10 BPH, 30 HSPC and 23 HRPC cancers. b) Illustration of Periostin expression (immunhistochemical data) in cancer-free patient samples (BPH) and invasive carcinomas (HSPC and HRPC).

5.5.7 Tissue inhibitor of metalloproteinase-1 (TMP-1) as a prognostic marker for survival of patients with hormone refractory prostate cancer (HRPC)

The proteins identified here could potentially serve different diagnostic purposes. Besides the early detection of prostate cancer, patient stratification and disease monitoring play important aspects[2]. PSA doubling time, the time required for PSA level to double, has been much advocated to monitor prostate cancer progression. However, PSA velocity, the change in PSA level over a specified time interval, added no predictive value to PSA level in either a study of long-term prediction of prostate cancer[33] or in the prostate cancer prevention trial (PCPT) study of biopsy outcome[34]. In order to test a few candidates for prognostic purposes, we have analyzed 32 patients with hormone refractory prostate cancer (HRPC) in respect to their serum levels of Carcinoembryonic antigen-related cell adhesion molecule 1 (CEACAM1), TSP-1, TIMP-1, PSA and PSA doubling time, respectively. As expected, PSA doubling time had no impact on patient's survival (p=0.583, log-rank test). Levels of CEACAM1, TSP-1 or PSA neither had any prognostic power. However, HRPC patients with TIMP-1 levels higher than 300 ng/ml had a much lower three-year survival rate (26.4%) compared to patients with lower serum levels of TIMP-1 (Figure 5.8). We also checked whether confounding factors could have led to this result. Conclusively neither age, body mass index (BMI) nor C-reactive protein (CPR) concentration and leukocyte number as indicators for inflammation correlated with TIMP-1 serum levels. TIMP-1 is not only known to inhibit matrix metalloproteinases but also to stimulate tumor growth. Several studies have shown that serum levels of TIMP-1 correlate with the long-term survival of patients with colorectal cancer[35] or breast cancer[36].

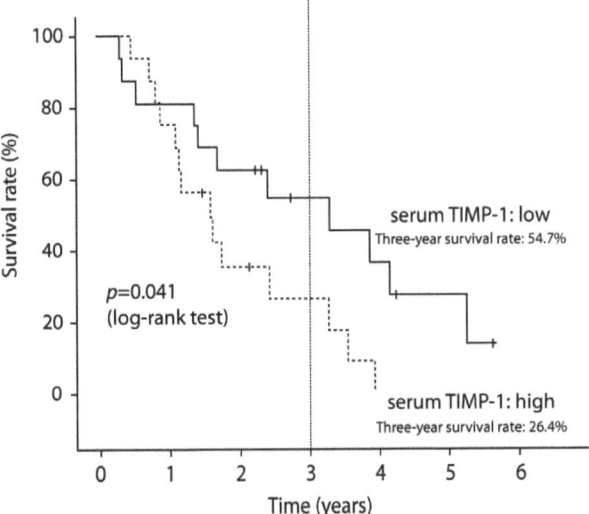

Figure 5.8 Survival curves in patients with high or low levels of tissue inhibitor of metalloproteinase-1 (TIMP-1).

5.6 Discussion

In this study we set out to find new biomarkers for the diagnosis of prostate cancer. Therefore, we employed a genetically engineered mouse model that reproduces the early steps of the human disease. In-depth analysis of the glyco-proteome in mouse tissues followed by the targeted analysis in mouse sera resulted in the identification of candidate markers. These proteins were then successfully monitored in blood samples of human patients resulting in a more accurate prediction of prostate cancer than currently available tests. Our findings here indicate that the use of mouse models in combination with in-depth quantitative MS analysis of glycoproteins and targeted MS thereof provides a useful strategy to identify candidate markers applicable to human cancer with potential utility for early detection.

Protein networks within proliferating cells regulate growth, division, maturation and survival. Genetic alterations can affect such protein networks and select towards robust and uncontrolled growth invasion of cancer cells. Here we have approached the problem of finding appropriate prostate cancer diagnostics by analyzing protein changes occurring upon PTEN-loss and downstream, constitutive PI3K/AKT pathway activation and consequent p53 activation. We have overcome the hurdle of artificial sample variations by employing a *Pten* cKO mouse model for prostate cancer, mimicking the early steps of human prostate cancer progression.

Comprehensive serum protein analysis is currently hampered by the high dynamic range of protein concentration and the few highly abundant serum proteins. In contrast, tissue is expected to reveal more meaningful disease related protein differences than serum because the challenges faced in serum are dramatically reduced. Especially protein concentration differences are expected to be more pronounced at the origin of the disease, than in the affected tissue itself. Thus, differential proteome profiles were directly investigated in the tissue of cancer-bearing and healthy mice. In fact, by simply comparing volumes of prostate tissue and blood, protein concentrations can be expected to be up to 1'000 fold higher in the tissue of origin, as compared to the same protein shed or secreted and diluted in the blood.

We focused our mass spectrometry (MS) based analysis on a very particular group of proteins, the glycoproteins. Glycoproteins are primarily present on the cell surface and are predominantly released through secretion and shedding into the bloodstream and therefore ideal diagnostic markers. Therefore we have employed a proteomics technology platform that allows for the selective isolation and quantification of glycoproteins from both tissue as well as from blood serum. Furthermore, the removal of high abundant non-glycoproteins facilitated the sensitive MS-based detection.

First, glycoprotein showing abundance differences among normal and cancer tissue were identified and later verified in the blood of the same mice. The human homologues of the discriminating mouse glycoproteins were validated in human patients by targeted mass spectrometry using SRM, a highly sensitive technology for protein quantification. The MS technology has three main advantages: (1) fast assay development and relatively cheap technology since no antibodies are needed as in the case of classical immunoassays. (2) Absolute quantification with the use of reference peptides. (3) High-

5 – Discovery and Validation of protein biomarkers for prostate cancer diagnosis

throughput measurement of up to 250 analytes per analysis. However, it has to be mentioned that yet SRM is not as sensitive and reproducible as a well-established ELISA. Nevertheless, targeted MS clearly is able to bridge the transition from marker candidate discovery to final validation by reducing the number of candidates through thorough verification.

Here we demonstrated that proteins originally detected in mouse tissue and verified in mouse serum represented valid marker candidates for diagnostic means in human prostate cancer patients. We compared blood serum samples from patients with BPH and locCaP. The reason for comparing these two patient groups is based on the fact that there are no precise tests for early prostate cancer detection, a disease that progresses mostly without symptoms to yet incurable metastases. Overdiagnosis of prostate cancer by PSA testing is a major problem in the clinics, as 75% of patients undergo unnecessary and painful biopsies and suffer from anxiety. Moreover, up to 10% of clinically relevant prostate cancers are not detected by PSA testing. To circumvent this unacceptable situation, a diagnostic test for prostate cancer is needed with higher specificity and sensitivity. Other clinical problems not yet solved can be as well addressed by our approach; such as the identification of markers that predict survival and therapeutic outcome of patients diagnosed with metastatic prostate cancer, a disease which is presently not curable. Conclusively, we unveiled a blood biomarker signature that can predicted localized prostate cancer more precisely with both higher sensitivity and specificity than PSA itself. Furthermore, Periostin was shown to be a valid tissue marker for the identification of metastatic cancer using IHC on biopsy specimens. We further showed that TIMP-1 concentration in the blood inversely correlated with future survival of patients with metastatic disease. Further validation efforts of potential biomarkers uncovered by our approach will thus not only lead to better diagnostic methods when compared to PSA but we will be able to address further questions that are yet to be solved in the clinics such as prediction of therapeutic outcome, diagnostic of defined genetic alterations and prediction of prostate cancer progression.

We identified a comprehensive catalog of glycoproteins of normal and cancer tissue and sera from a genetically defined mouse model of prostate cancer. A further highly relevant application of our screen relies on the identification of therapeutic targets. The glycoproteins located on the cell surface that quantitatively changed during tumor progression represent indeed potential novel targets for the development of anti-cancer agents. These potential targets are currently tested and prioritized using TMA, bioinformatic analysis as well as functional cell based assays (RNAi screening) to test whether stimulation or inhibition of such targets leads to the dead or proliferative senescence of cultured prostate cancer cells. The MS-based analysis of the *in vivo* *N*-linked glyco-proteome from genetically defined mice thus is a suitable approach to address multiple and highly relevant clinical questions for the detection, prediction and therapy of human cancers.

5.7 References

1. Jemal, A. et al. Cancer statistics, 2007. *CA Cancer J Clin* **57**, 43-66 (2007).
2. Lilja, H., Ulmert, D. & Vickers, A.J. Prostate-specific antigen and prostate cancer: prediction, detection and monitoring. *Nat Rev Cancer* **8**, 268-78 (2008).
3. Cully, M., You, H., Levine, A. & Mak, T. Beyond PTEN mutations: the PI3K pathway as an integrator of multiple inputs during tumorigenesis. *Nat Rev Cancer* **6**, 184-92 (2006).
4. Trotman, L.C. et al. Pten dose dictates cancer progression in the prostate. *PLoS Biol* **1**, E59 (2003).
5. Wu, X., Senechal, K., Neshat, M.S., Whang, Y.E. & Sawyers, C.L. The PTEN/MMAC1 tumor suppressor phosphatase functions as a negative regulator of the phosphoinositide 3-kinase/Akt pathway. *Proc Natl Acad Sci USA* **95**, 15587-91 (1998).
6. Zhang, H., Li, X.J., Martin, D.B. & Aebersold, R.H. Identification and quantification of N-linked glycoproteins using hydrazide chemistry, stable isotope labeling and mass spectrometry. *Nat Biotechnol* **21**, 660-6 (2003).
7. Pedrioli, P.G. et al. A common open representation of mass spectrometry data and its application to proteomics research. *Nat Biotechnol* **22**, 1459-66 (2004).
8. Eng, J.K., McCormack, A.L. & Yates, J.R. An approach to correlate tandem mass spectral data of peptides with amino acid sequences in a protein database. *J Am Soc Mass Spectrom* **5**, 976-89 (1994).
9. Keller, A., Eng, J.K., Zhang, N., Li, X.J. & Aebersold, R.H. A uniform proteomics MS/MS analysis platform utilizing open XML file formats. *Mol Syst Biol* **1**, 2005.0017 (2005).
10. Keller, A., Nesvizhskii, A.I., Kolker, E. & Aebersold, R.H. Empirical statistical model to estimate the accuracy of peptide identifications made by MS/MS and database search. *Anal Chem* **74**, 5383-92 (2002).
11. Nesvizhskii, A.I., Keller, A., Kolker, E. & Aebersold, R.H. A statistical model for identifying proteins by tandem mass spectrometry. *Anal Chem* **75**, 4646-58 (2003).
12. Mueller, L.N. et al. SuperHirn - a novel tool for high resolution LC-MS-based peptide/protein profiling. *Proteomics* **7**, 3470-80 (2007).
13. Schiess, R. et al. Analysis of cell surface proteome changes via label-free, quantitative mass spectrometry. *Mol Cell Proteomics* **8**, 624-38 (2009).
14. Theurillat, J.P. et al. Distinct expression patterns of the immunogenic differentiation antigen NY-BR-1 in normal breast, testis and their malignant counterparts. *Int J Cancer* **122**, 1585-91 (2008).
15. Gerber, S.A., Rush, J., Stemman, O., Kirschner, M.W. & Gygi, S.P. Absolute quantification of proteins and phosphoproteins from cell lysates by tandem MS. *Proc Natl Acad Sci USA* **100**, 6940-5 (2003).
16. Lange, V. et al. Targeted quantitative analysis of Streptococcus pyogenes virulence factors by multiple reaction monitoring. *Mol Cell Proteomics* (2008).
17. Vlietstra, R.J., van Alewijk, D.C., Hermans, K.G., van Steenbrugge, G.J. & Trapman, J. Frequent inactivation of PTEN in prostate cancer cell lines and xenografts. *Cancer Res* **58**, 2720-3 (1998).
18. DeMarzo, A.M., Nelson, W.G., Isaacs, W.B. & Epstein, J.I. Pathological and molecular aspects of prostate cancer. *Lancet* **361**, 955-64 (2003).
19. Vivanco, I. & Sawyers, C.L. The phosphatidylinositol 3-Kinase AKT pathway in human cancer. *Nat Rev Cancer* **2**, 489-501 (2002).
20. Liu, H., Sadygov, R.G. & Yates, J.R. A model for random sampling and estimation of relative protein abundance in shotgun proteomics. *Anal Chem* **76**, 4193-201 (2004).
21. Ishihama, Y. et al. Exponentially modified protein abundance index (emPAI) for estimation of absolute protein amount in proteomics by the number of sequenced peptides per protein. *Mol Cell Proteomics* **4**, 1265-72 (2005).
22. Su, A.I. et al. Large-scale analysis of the human and mouse transcriptomes. *Proc Natl Acad Sci USA* **99**, 4465-70 (2002).
23. Wen, S. et al. PTEN controls tumor-induced angiogenesis. *Proc Natl Acad Sci USA* **98**, 4622-7 (2001).
24. Dameron, K.M., Volpert, O.V., Tainsky, M.A. & Bouck, N. Control of angiogenesis in fibroblasts by p53 regulation of thrombospondin-1. *Science* **265**, 1582-4 (1994).
25. Chen, Z. et al. Crucial role of p53-dependent cellular senescence in suppression of Pten-deficient tumorigenesis. *Nature* **436**, 725-30 (2005).
26. Patrawala, L. et al. Highly purified CD44+ prostate cancer cells from xenograft human tumors are enriched in tumorigenic and metastatic progenitor cells. *Oncogene* **25**, 1696-708 (2006).
27. Doll, J.A. et al. Thrombospondin-1, vascular endothelial growth factor and fibroblast growth factor-2 are key functional regulators of angiogenesis in the prostate. *Prostate* **49**, 293-305 (2001).
28. Payne, S.L., Hendrix, M.J. & Kirschmann, D.A. Paradoxical roles for lysyl oxidases in cancer--a prospect. *J Cell Biochem* **101**, 1338-54 (2007).
29. Stefansson, S. & Lawrence, D.A. The serpin PAI-1 inhibits cell migration by blocking integrin alpha V beta 3 binding to vitronectin. *Nature* **383**, 441-3 (1996).
30. Turashvili, G. et al. Novel markers for differentiation of lobular and ductal invasive breast carcinomas by laser microdissection and microarray analysis. *BMC Cancer* **7**, 55 (2007).

5 – Discovery and validation of protein biomarkers for prostate cancer diagnosis

31. Kudo, Y., Siriwardena, B.S., Hatano, H., Ogawa, I. & Takata, T. Periostin: novel diagnostic and therapeutic target for cancer. *Histol Histopathol* **22**, 1167-74 (2007).
32. Kristiansen, G. et al. GOLPH2 protein expression as a novel tissue biomarker for prostate cancer: implications for tissue-based diagnostics. *Br J Cancer* **99**, 939-48 (2008).
33. Ulmert, D. et al. Long-term prediction of prostate cancer: prostate-specific antigen (PSA) velocity is predictive but does not improve the predictive accuracy of a single PSA measurement 15 years or more before cancer diagnosis in a large, representative, unscreened population. *J Clin Oncol* **26**, 835-41 (2008).
34. Thompson, I.M. et al. Assessing prostate cancer risk: results from the Prostate Cancer Prevention Trial. *J Natl Cancer Inst* **98**, 529-34 (2006).
35. Yukawa, N. et al. Impact of plasma tissue inhibitor of matrix metalloproteinase-1 on long-term survival in patients with colorectal cancer. *Oncology* **72**, 205-8 (2007).
36. Schrohl, A.S. et al. Tumor tissue levels of tissue inhibitor of metalloproteinase-1 as a prognostic marker in primary breast cancer. *Clin Cancer Res* **10**, 2289-98 (2004).

6 Summary of results

The goal of my thesis was to elaborate a new proteomic strategy for the successful identification and validation of proteins for diagnostic purposes. Many diseases such as cancer are highly dependant on the early diagnosis and thus their prevention because late stage diseases are more difficult to cure. Diagnostic markers are not only thought to prevent disease, but also to monitor treatment and to assist the development of new therapeutics. Current protein biomarker discovery strategies are mainly limited by the low sample reproducibility from patient to patient and the large dynamic range of protein concentrations. In order to overcome these difficulties, I decided to mainly focus and thereby improving the following crucial steps:

Firstly, in order to be able to identify *N*-glycosites and *O*-glycosites from potential protein biomarker candidates, I developed a strategy for the specific enrichment and subsequent multiplexed identification of *O*-glycosites, which can be coupled to the well-established isolation of *N*-glycosites. To achieve this goal I initially optimized successfully the reaction conditions for the chemical release of *O*-linked glycans from peptides. By using the optimized reaction conditions in combination with a modified workflow for the selective enrichment of both *N*- and *O*-glycosites, I was able to show the feasibility of this approach in experiments resulting in the combined proteomic identification of *N*- and *O*-glycosites from a model glycoprotein. Subsequently, I applied the dual strategy to a complex mixture of blood serum glycoproteins showing the combined identification of *N*- and *O*-linked glycopeptides. This approach led to new *O*-glycosite containing protein identifications, which is a so far mostly uncharted territory. The presented approach therefore has the ability to extend the current mostly *N*-glycosite-based glyco-proteome coverage.

Secondly, I was involved in developing a methodology for the multiplexed, quantitative, mass-spectrometric identification of cell surface glycoproteins, which can be used to phenotype cells without antibodies, in an unbiased fashion, and without *a priori* knowledge. The cell surface capturing (CSC) technology allows for the isolation, identification and quantification of *N*-glycosites from the extracellular domains of cell surface proteins in a discovery-driven mode. Several hundred *bona fide* cell surface glycoproteins and their *N*-glycosites, including CD-annotated and novel proteins, could be identified in a single MS experiment. I could specifically show that the CSC technology is highly reproducible in *Drosophila melanogaster* cell experiments and that the approach is not dependent on terminal sialic acid residues.

Thirdly, I combined the CSC technology with new label-free MS-based quantification technologies in order to be able to detect dynamic cell surface proteome changes. The strategy is based on the label-free quantification of peptide patterns acquired by high mass accuracy mass spectrometry. The strategy was applied to monitor dynamic protein changes in the cell surface glyco-proteome of *D. melanogaster* cells. The results led to the construction of a cell surface glycoprotein atlas consisting of 202 cell surface glycoproteins of *D. melanogaster* Kc167 cells indicating relative quantitative changes of cell surface glycoproteins in four different cellular states. Furthermore, I specifically investigated cell surface proteome changes upon prolonged insulin stimulation. The data revealed insulin-dependent cell surface glycoprotein dynamics, including insulin receptor internalization, and linked these changes to intracellular signaling networks.

Finally, I developed and applied an integrated strategy for the MS-based identification and quantification of glycoprotein biomarker candidates from minute amounts of blood. The strategy is based on the assumption that tissue derived proteins specific for a particular disease can be detected in the blood. In a Pten conditional knock-out (cKO) mouse model for prostate cancer progression I performed a quantitative comparison of the glycoprotein profile from Pten cKO prostate cancer and control tissue. My experiments revealed a panel of differently expressed biomarker candidate glycoproteins in tissue. A subset of these glycoproteins was then monitored in the blood of the Pten cKO mouse model by using absolute quantitative SRM at different time points. Accordingly, we sought to explore the merits of the genetically defined Pten cKO model of prostate cancer to determine whether such changes are relevant to human prostate cancer. The experiments showed that a three glycoprotein signature in combination with PSA predicted localized prostate cancer in men more precisely than currently available tests. Furthermore, these results show that a strategy combining the use of a mouse model with in-depth quantitative MS analysis of glycoproteins and subsequent targeted MS analysis of biomarker candidates is applicable to the identification of biomarkers for human cancer.

7 Conclusions

Cancer is one of the leading causes of mortality in developed countries. It affects people of all ages, but most cancers are detected in people aged 55 or older. One out of two men and one out of three women are statistically expected to develop cancer within their lifetime. Since lifetime expectancy is continuously rising early cancer diagnosis is gaining attention because the accurate and timely detection of diseases in general is expected to result in a better chance for patient survival and reduced health costs for the society. However, most of today's protein-based early diagnostic screening methods are still in their infancy and lack sensitivity and specificity or are dependent on available protein-specific antibodies. The mass spectrometry (MS) assisted discovery, verification and validation strategy presented here indicates now a new approach towards the sensitive and selective early detection of disease classifying biomarkers circumventing the above mentioned problems to a large extent.

The technologies developed, and the approach for biomarker discovery chosen here in this PhD thesis indicate new ways of addressing the problem of how to identify protein panels for the early detection of cancer (Figure 7.1). Most MS-based proteomic biomarker discovery efforts focus on blood profiling of patients and healthy individuals. Due to the enormous complexity of the blood proteome and the large variations among the blood samples collected only limited success was achieved so far. Here I focused on the comparison of disease affected and control tissue proteomes to overcome sensitivity issues. Furthermore an animal model was employed to reduce sample heterogeneity and to study disease relevant changes that could be specifically engineered using the mouse model employed here. Another important point of the strategy applied was the focus on the glyco-proteome. The selective enrichment and quantitative analysis of glycoproteins not only reduced the sample complexity, but also proofed to be a subproteome of great interest in respect to protein biomarkers. Since a major part of the glycoproteins are secreted, shed or otherwise released by the cell the systematic analysis of this important subproteome therefore opens the possibility of detecting molecular signatures in body fluids indicating the state of a cell or tissue. The analysis of glycoproteins was thus ideally suited for the detection of such sets of proteins in the patient's blood in a non-invasive manner.

Currently, the lack of further verification of proteins identified in proteomic screens for biomarkers is a huge limitation. Antibody-based assays cannot fill this obvious gap due to their long and expensive generation time. The usage of targeted MS using selected reaction monitoring (SRM) allowed us for the subsequent verification of candidate markers in murine blood followed by the validation in human patients of interesting biomarker candidates. SRM is a highly sensitive technology for protein quantification. In contrast to antibody-based technologies such as ELISA, SRM assays can be relatively quickly established at low cost. Moreover, the usage of reference peptides enables absolute quantification. However, it has to be realized that yet SRM is not as sensitive and reproducible as a well-established ELISA. Nevertheless, we demonstrated the reproducible measurement of proteins in blood serum at as low as single digit ng/ml concentrations. While up to 250 analytes can be simultaneously measured per analysis, sample throughput is limited to one sample per hour. This makes SRM the ideal method to be applied for the verification of hundreds of potential biomarkers in order to bridge the initial discovery and clinical validation phases. The results presented clearly demonstrated the feasibility of the suggested strategy for biomarker discovery, verification and validation as illustrated in Figure 7.1.

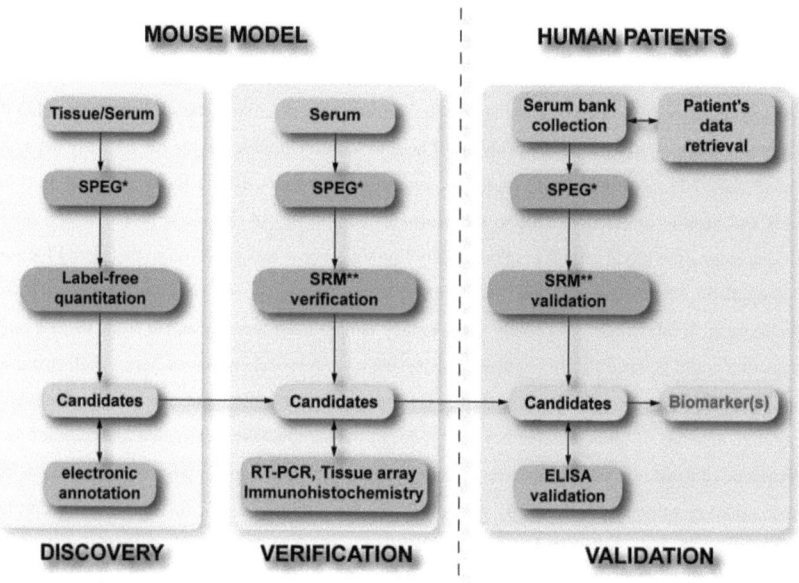

SPEG*: Solid-Phase Extraction of Glycopeptides
SRM**: Selected Reaction Monitoring

Figure 7.1 Integrated proteomics strategy for the discovery, verification and validation of protein biomarkers. Glycoproteins are specifically enriched from mouse tissue and blood serum using solid-phase extraction of glycoproteins (SPEG) and quantified by label-free comparison of healthy and diseased samples. Interesting proteins are then verified in blood serum by targeted MS using selected reaction monitoring (SRM) at high specificity and sensitivity. Additionally, real-time PCR, tissue microarray (TMA) and IHC based experiments are carried out for further indications. Finally, potential protein biomarkers are measured in human patients by SRM and if available by ELISA to identify statistically significant protein signatures that identify disease affected patients.

7 – Conclusions

Due to its appealing properties to biomarker discovery, I set out to extend the glyco-proteome coverage to O-linked glycoproteins. In contrast to the well-established enzymatic release of solid-phase enriched N-glycopeptides, the release of O-glycopeptides was problematic due to the lack of an efficient enzymatic strategy. Here, I presented a chemical strategy for the concurrent identification of N- and O-linked glycoproteins, which will be implemented into further glyco-proteome-based biomarker discovery research.

Cell surface proteins are carrying out various important functions and are therefore important targets in many pharmacological studies. We have developed a robust, MS-based technology for the multiplexed identification and quantification of cell surface glycoproteins. It is ideally suited for multiplexed, discovery-driven identification and quantification of cell surface glycoproteins. I demonstrated its combination with label-free quantification and showed that specific proteomic fingerprints could be assigned indicating a cells origin, function and physical state using our proteomics and informatics pipeline. Cell surface proteins are not only interesting diagnostic but also therapeutic targets. Their accessibility on the cell surface makes them ideal targets for inhibitors such as small molecules or antibodies. The research efforts presented here identified various interesting proteins such as GPCRs, receptor tyrosine kinases, proteases, etc. that could be potential drugable targets.

Conclusively, the strategy presented has the potential to identify both diagnostic markers and therapeutic targets. As the health care system is shifting to personalized medicine, diagnostic and therapy can no longer be considered as two separate entities. Diagnostic markers are needed for the development of new drugs in order to have valid control mechanisms, which adds additional safety constraints, identifies patient target groups, defines valid dosage and endpoints of studies. For these reasons it can be expected in the near future that drug agencies will request valid biomarkers for drug development. Furthermore, there is a great demand for a well-established diagnostic and therapeutic interplay in daily clinical practice where disease management is greatly dependant on prognostic, stratification and efficacy markers.

Supplemental Material

Supplementary Table S2.1 List of O- and N-linked glycoproteins. The list comprises all glycoproteins identified in blood serum using the combined strategy for O- and N-glycoprotein enrichment. The following SEQUEST score cutoffs were used: Xcorr > 2.5, ΔC_n > 0.1, and SpRank < 5 (applied to all peptide charge states). Displayed columns include the IPI ID (Human v3.36); UniProt AC; Protein name; glycosylation status.

IPI identifier	UniProt AC	Protein Name	Glycosylation status
IPI00022431	P02765	Alpha-2-HS-glycoprotein (Fetuin-A)	O-, N-linked
IPI00022488	P02790	Hemopexin (Beta-1B-glycoprotein).	O-, N-linked
IPI00291866	P05155	Plasma protease C1 inhibitor	O-, N-linked
IPI00550991	P01011	Alpha-1-antichymotrypsin precursor (ACT)	O-, N-linked
IPI00014072	O96017	Serine/threonine-protein kinase Chk2	O-linked
IPI00020546	Q9NR48	Probable histone-lysine N-methyltransferase ASH1L	O-linked
IPI00022426	P02760	AMBP protein	O-linked
IPI00029011	O60333	Kinesin-like protein KIF1B (Klp)	O-linked
IPI00083708	Q05DM8	Hypothetical protein	O-linked
IPI00103552	Q8WXI7	Mucin-16, Ovarian carcinoma antigen CA125 (CA-125)	O-linked
IPI00221325	P49742	E3 SUMO-protein ligase RanBP2	O-linked
IPI00296942	P55289	Cadherin-12	O-linked
IPI00297859	O14686	Myeloid/lymphoid or mixed-lineage leukemia protein 2	O-linked
IPI00005024	Q9BQG0	Myb-binding protein 1A	O-linked
IPI00007957	Q9Y6J9	PCAF-associated factor 65 alpha (PAF65- alpha)	O-linked
IPI00009319	Q9NZQ3	SH3 adapter protein SPIN90	O-linked
IPI00016177	Q99583	Max-binding protein MNT	O-linked
IPI00018429	Q99811	Paired mesoderm homeobox protein 2	O-linked
IPI00019848	P51610	Host cell factor (HCF)	O-linked
IPI00021857	P02656	Apolipoprotein C-III precursor (Apo-CIII)	O-linked
IPI00032358	Q9Y2N3	Nuclear envelope pore membrane protein POM 121	O-linked
IPI00042612	Q9BUU2	C16orf68 protein	O-linked
IPI00064798	Q96KT6	Uncharacterized protein C8orf14	O-linked
IPI00103397	Q8WWQ5	Mucin 5	O-linked
IPI00107122	Q9BVL2	Nucleoporin p58/p45	O-linked
IPI00217244	Q8IWA6	Coiled-coil domain-containing protein 60	O-linked
IPI00291624	Q8WXF0	35 kDa SR repressor protein	O-linked
IPI00294958	O75112	LIM domain-binding protein 3	O-linked
IPI00303075	Q6UW49	Sperm equatorial segment protein 1	O-linked
IPI00328253	P78415	Iroquois-class homeodomain protein IRX-3	O-linked
IPI00383270	Q14888	Mucin	O-linked
IPI00384775	O14760	Small intestinal mucin MUC3	O-linked
IPI00386766	Q02505	Mucin-3A (Intestinal mucin-3A)	O-linked
IPI00398971	Q7L530	FLJ30092 protein	O-linked
IPI00401759	A2A329	Family with sequence similarity 102, member A	O-linked
IPI00401776	Q6W4X9	Mucin-6 (Gastric mucin-6)	O-linked
IPI00410480	Q6ZUA9	CDNA FLJ43860 fis, clone TESTI4007404	O-linked
IPI00419247	NA	37 kDa protein	O-linked
IPI00452590	Q8IWK6	Probable G-protein coupled receptor 125	O-linked
IPI00454767	A8MXV8	Uncharacterized protein ENSP00000381951	O-linked
IPI00549566	Q5T160	Probable arginyl-tRNA synthetase	O-linked
IPI00645765	O95226	Voltage-gated L-type calcium channel alpha-1 subunit	O-linked
IPI00737498	Q9H8R3	CDNA FLJ13298 fis, clone OVARC1001306	O-linked
IPI00807694	Q711P9	Uncharacterized protein C10orf471	O-linked
IPI00829826	B2RAG9	cDNA, FLJ94908	O-linked
IPI00855918	Q9HC84	Mucin-5B	O-linked
IPI00868729	NA	Similar to ELK1 protein	O-linked
IPI00871194	NA	Uncharacterized protein ENSP00000380619	O-linked
IPI00872675	NA	Uncharacterized protein ENSP00000383218	O-linked
IPI00874244	Q69YU0	Putative uncharacterized protein DKFZp547N024	O-linked
IPI00006114	P36955	Pigment epithelium-derived factor precursor (PEDF)	N-linked
IPI00006154	P36980	Complement factor H-related protein 2	N-linked
IPI00006662	P05090	Apolipoprotein D	N-linked
IPI00007221	P05154	Plasma serine protease inhibitor	N-linked
IPI00007240	P05160	Coagulation factor XIII B chain	N-linked
IPI00009793	Q53GX9	Complement C1r-like protein	N-linked
IPI00013179	P41222	Prostaglandin-H2 D-isomerase	N-linked
IPI00017601	P00450	Ceruloplasmin	N-linked
IPI00017696	P09871	Complement C1s subcomponent	N-linked
IPI00018305	P17936	Insulin-like growth factor-binding protein 3	N-linked

IPI identifier	UniProt AC	Protein Name	Glycosylation status
IPI00019568	P00734	Prothrombin	N-linked
IPI00019581	P00748	Coagulation factor XII	N-linked
IPI00019591	P00751	Complement factor B	N-linked
IPI00019943	P43652	Afamin	N-linked
IPI00020091	P19652	Alpha-1-acid glycoprotein 2	N-linked
IPI00020986	P51884	Lumican	N-linked
IPI00020996	P35858	Insulin-like growth factor-binding protein	N-linked
IPI00021727	P04003	C4b-binding protein alpha chain	N-linked
IPI00022229	P04114	Apolipoprotein B-100	N-linked
IPI00022371	P04196	Histidine-rich glycoprotein	N-linked
IPI00022395	P02748	Complement component C9	N-linked
IPI00022418	P02751	Fibronectin	N-linked
IPI00022429	P02763	Alpha-1-acid glycoprotein 1	N-linked
IPI00022463	P02787	Serotransferrin	N-linked
IPI00022895	P04217	Alpha-1B-glycoprotein	N-linked
IPI00023019	P04278	Sex hormone-binding globulin	N-linked
IPI00023246	Q92748	Thyroid hormone-inducible hepatic protein	N-linked
IPI00023673	Q08380	Galectin-3-binding protein	N-linked
IPI00025862	P20851	C4b-binding protein beta chain	N-linked
IPI00025864	P06276	Cholinesterase	N-linked
IPI00027235	O75882	Attractin	N-linked
IPI00027482	P08185	Corticosteroid-binding globulin	N-linked
IPI00029061	P49908	Selenoprotein P	N-linked
IPI00029739	P08603	Complement factor H	N-linked
IPI00029863	P08697	Alpha-2-antiplasmin	N-linked
IPI00032179	Q7KZ97	Antithrombin III variant.	N-linked
IPI00032220	P01019	Angiotensinogen	N-linked
IPI00032258	P0C0L4	Complement C4-A	N-linked
IPI00032328	P01042	Kininogen-1	N-linked
IPI00061977	Q9BRV0	IGHA1 protein.	N-linked
IPI00103419	Q8IWZ8	Splicing factor 4	N-linked
IPI00163207	Q96PD5	N-acetylmuramoyl-L-alanine amidase	N-linked
IPI00166533	Q1XH10	DLN-1.	N-linked
IPI00166729	P25311	Zinc-alpha-2-glycoprotein	N-linked
IPI00168728	Q8NF17	FLJ00385 protein (Fragment).	N-linked
IPI00218192	Q14624	Inter-alpha-trypsin inhibitor heavy chain H4	N-linked
IPI00218413	P43251	Biotinidase	N-linked
IPI00218732	P27169	Serum paraoxonase/arylesterase 1	N-linked
IPI00218795	P14151	L-selectin	N-linked
IPI00291262	P10909	Clusterin	N-linked
IPI00292946	P05543	Thyroxine-binding globulin	N-linked
IPI00293057	Q96IY4	Carboxypeptidase B2	N-linked
IPI00294004	P07225	Vitamin K-dependent protein S	N-linked
IPI00294395	P07358	Complement component C8 beta chain	N-linked
IPI00298828	P02749	Beta-2-glycoprotein 1	N-linked
IPI00298971	P04004	Vitronectin	N-linked
IPI00303963	P06681	Complement C2	N-linked
IPI00305461	P19823	Inter-alpha-trypsin inhibitor heavy chain H2	N-linked
IPI00328609	P29622	Kallistatin	N-linked
IPI00382606	Q96PQ8	Factor VII active site mutant immunoconjugate	N-linked
IPI00384952	Q7Z379	Hypothetical protein DKFZp686K04218	N-linked
IPI00385264	P04220	Ig mu heavy chain disease protein	N-linked
IPI00386797	Q9BUT0	FNIP1 protein	N-linked
IPI00013302	Q13444	ADAM 15	N-linked
IPI00019376	Q9NVA2	Septin-11	N-linked
IPI00023532	Q9NTW4	SPATS2-like protein	N-linked
IPI00157414	Q6UWR7	Ectonucleotide pyrophosphatase/phosphodiesterase 6	N-linked
IPI00167609	Q8N961	Ankyrin repeat and BTB/POZ domain-containing protein 2	N-linked
IPI00173549	B2RWP6	Synaptopodin 2	N-linked
IPI00217512	Q8IZF3	G-protein coupled receptor PGR18	N-linked
IPI00251161	Q9H742	CDNA: FLJ21404 fis, clone COL03835	N-linked
IPI00384391	Q9UL71	Myosin-reactive immunoglobulin	N-linked
IPI00431645	Q6NSB4	HP protein	N-linked
IPI00478003	P01023	Alpha-2-macroglobulin	N-linked
IPI00478539	NA	Similar to heterogeneous nuclear ribonucleoprotein A1	N-linked
IPI00479116	P22792	Carboxypeptidase N subunit 2	N-linked
IPI00552199	Q5J876	GUGU beta form	N-linked
IPI00553177	P01009	Alpha-1-antitrypsin precursor	N-linked
IPI00555909	Q569H4	Proline-rich protein 16	N-linked
IPI00654888	Q17RE8	Kallikrein B	N-linked
IPI00783987	P01024	Complement C3	N-linked
IPI00785036	Q68CJ6	Hypothetical protein HMFN0672	N-linked
IPI00869111	NA	Similar to Phosducin-like protein 3	N-linked
IPI00880053	B3GQS7	Mitochondrial heat shock 60kD protein 1 variant 1	N-linked

Supplemental Material

Supplementary Table S2.2 List of O-linked glycoproteins including their site of modification. The list comprises all O-linked glycoproteins identified in blood serum using the combined strategy for O- and N-glycoprotein enrichment. The following SEQUEST score cutoffs were used: Xcorr > 2.5, ΔC_n > 0.1, and SpRank < 5 (applied to all peptide charge states). Displayed columns include the IPI ID (Human v3.36); UniProt AC; Protein name; glycosylation site.

IPI identifier	UniProt Accession	Protein Name	Glycosylation site
IPI00005024	Q9BQG0	Myb-binding protein 1A	T961, S967, S983, T987
IPI00007957	Q9Y6J9	PCAF-associated factor 65 alpha (PAF65- alpha)	S501, S521
IPI00009319	Q9NZQ3	SH3 adapter protein SPIN90	S197, S199
IPI00014072	O96017	Serine/threonine-protein kinase Chk2	S24, T26, S32, S49
IPI00016177	Q99583	Max-binding protein MNT	T567, S577, T578
IPI00018429	Q99811	Paired mesoderm homeobox protein 2	S205, S206, S218, T223
IPI00019848	P51610	Host cell factor (HCF)	S806, T816, T831
IPI00020546	Q9NR48	Probable histone-lysine N-methyltransferase ASH1L	S2330, S2334, T2339
IPI00021857	P02656	Apolipoprotein C-III precursor (Apo-CIII)	T94
IPI00022426	P02760	AMBP protein	S215
IPI00022431	P02765	Alpha-2-HS-glycoprotein (Fetuin-A)	S280, S347
IPI00022488	P02790	Hemopexin (Beta-1B-glycoprotein).	T29
IPI00029011	O60333	Kinesin-like protein KIF1B (Klp)	T1439
IPI00032358	Q9Y2N3	Nuclear envelope pore membrane protein POM 121	T1139, T1148, T1149, S1151
IPI00042612	Q9BUU2	C16orf68 protein	S68, T74, T85
IPI00064798	Q96KT6	Uncharacterized protein C8orf14	S70, T78
IPI00083708	Q05DM8	Hypothetical protein	S1812, S1816, S1818
IPI00103397	Q8WWQ5	Mucin 5	T2314, T2329, T2330, S2331
IPI00103552	Q8WXI7	Mucin-16, Ovarian carcinoma antigen CA125 (CA-125)	S2365, T2376, S2380, S2381
IPI00107122	Q9BVL2	Nucleoporin p58/p45	S70, T91, T94, T97
IPI00217244	Q8IWA6	Coiled-coil domain-containing protein 60	S245
IPI00221325	P49792	E3 SUMO-protein ligase RanBP2	S1884, T1885, S1903
IPI00291624	Q8WXF0	35 kDa SR repressor protein	S224, S235, T241
IPI00291866	P05155	Plasma protease C1 inhibitor	S28, S150, S158
IPI00294958	O75112	LIM domain-binding protein 3	T98, S110, S112
IPI00296942	P55289	Cadherin-12	S744, S746, S750, T769
IPI00297859	O14686	Myeloid/lymphoid or mixed-lineage leukemia protein 2	S3021, S3030, S3039
IPI00303075	Q6UW49	Sperm equatorial segment protein 1	S179, T183, S187, T188
IPI00328253	P78415	Iroquois-class homeodomain protein IRX-3	S288, S291
IPI00383270	Q14888	Mucin	T72, T73, S79, T80, S82, T88, T94
IPI00384775	O14760	Small intestinal mucin MUC3	S238, T249, S271, T273
IPI00386766	Q02505	Mucin-3A (Intestinal mucin-3A)	S1156, T1162, S1181, T1184
IPI00398971	Q7L530	FLJ30092 protein	S217, S223
IPI00401759	A2A329	Family with sequence similarity 102, member A	S105, S126, T132
IPI00401776	Q6W4X9	Mucin-6 (Gastric mucin-6)	S1944, T1955, S1956, S1960
IPI00410480	Q6ZUA9	CDNA FLJ43860 fis, clone TESTI4007404	S940, S942, S950, T954
IPI00419247	NA	37 kDa protein	S278, S284, S291, S304
IPI00452590	Q8IWK6	Probable G-protein coupled receptor 125	T247, S249, S259
IPI00454977	A8MXV8	Uncharacterized protein ENSP00000381951	T265
IPI00549566	Q5T160	Probable arginyl-tRNA synthetase	S309, S316, T319, S320
IPI00550991	P01011	Alpha-1-antichymotrypsin precursor (ACT)	T135
IPI00645765	O95226	Voltage-gated L-type calcium channel alpha-1 subunit	S4, S15, T18
IPI00737298	Q9H8R3	CDNA FLJ13298 fis, clone OVARC1001306	S1679, T1682, S1695
IPI00807694	Q711P9	Uncharacterized protein C10orf71	S81, T84, T95
IPI00829826	B2RAG9	cDNA, FLJ94908	S1229, S1240, S1247, S1254
IPI00855918	Q9HC84	Mucin-5B	T2609, S2624, S2626, T2632
IPI00868729	NA	Similar to ELK1 protein	S80, S83, S94
IPI00871194	NA	Uncharacterized protein ENSP00000380619	S231, T234, S254, S259
IPI00872675	NA	Uncharacterized protein ENSP00000383218	S143, T155
IPI00874244	Q69YU0	Putative uncharacterized protein DKFZp547N024	S8

Supplementary Table S3.1 CSC identified Jurkat T lymphocyte proteins. MS identified proteins from Jurkat T lymphocytes by using the CSC technology. Shown is the list of 110 protein identifications, including 43 CD proteins, with a ProteinProphet probability of 0.9 or higher. The specificity for CSC proteins is 95%. The proteins were identified from one experimental sample which was run back to back two times under the same conditions on an LTQ-FT. The sample was run twice for statistical purposes in order to increase the confidence in the peptide identifications. Displayed columns include the IPI ID (Human v3.26); UniProt AC; Protein name; ProteinProphet probability (PP); the number of uniquely identified peptides/protein; the total number of identified peptides/protein; CD annotation; SOSUI and TMHMM transmembrane prediction.

IPI ID	UniProt AC	Protein Name	PP	num unique peps	tot num peps	CD	Sosui TM	TM HMM
IPI00000877	Q9Y4L1	150 kDa oxygen-regulated protein.	1.00	2	5		1	1
IPI00002478	P42892	Isoform B of endothelin-converting enzyme 1.	1.00	2	3		1	1
IPI00003648	Q15223	Isoform delta of poliovirus receptor-related protein 1.	1.00	4	16	CD111	2	2
IPI00003813	A0A4Z1	Nectin-like protein 2.	1.00	4	23		2	1
IPI00006071	P28907	Isoform 1 of ADP-ribosyl cyclase 1.	1.00	3	8	CD38	1	1
IPI00009477	P13598	Intercellular adhesion molecule 2.	1.00	15	74	CD102	2	1
IPI00009803	P13612	Integrin alpha-4.	1.00	4	9	CD49d	2	1
IPI00011578	Q9Y639	Isoform 1 of neuroplastin.	1.00	4	21		2	1
IPI00012977	O00478	Butyrophilin subfamily 3 member A3.	1.00	2	4		1	1
IPI00013831	P09326	Cd48 antigen.	1.00	5	25	CD48	2	1
IPI00014236	Q15043	Solute carrier family 39 member 14.	1.00	3	5		4	6
IPI00014854	Q07108	Early activation antigen CD69.	1.00	3	11	CD69	1	1
IPI00015199	P09564	T-cell antigen CD7.	1.00	3	8	CD7	2	1
IPI00015476	P43007	Neutral amino acid transporter a.	1.00	5	14		9	9
IPI00019906	P35613	Isoform 2 of basigin.	1.00	10	54	CD147	2	2
IPI00021058	Q9Y6M7	Isoform 3 of sodium bicarbonate cotransporter 3.	1.00	5	15		11	11
IPI00022462	P02786	Transferrin receptor protein 1.	1.00	4	16	CD71	1	1
IPI00022649	P55011	Isoform 1 of solute carrier family 12 member 2.	1.00	2	5		11	12
IPI00022892	P04216	Thy-1 membrane glycoprotein.	1.00	5	20	CD90	2	0
IPI00023807	Q92854	Semaphorin-4d.	1.00	7	28	CD100	2	2
IPI00023814	Q92859	Isoform 1 of neogenin.	1.00	3	9		2	1
IPI00026241	Q10589	Bone marrow stromal antigen 2.	1.00	2	6	CD317	1	1
IPI00027493	P08195	4F2 cell-surface antigen heavy chain.	1.00	22	112	CD98	1	1
IPI00027505	P06756	Integrin alpha-v.	1.00	2	8	CD51	2	1
IPI00027728	P30825	High-affinity cationic amino acid transporter 1.	1.00	4	13		14	14
IPI00028015	Q6GTX8	Leukocyte-associated immunoglobulin-like receptor 1.	1.00	2	12	CD305	2	1
IPI00028931	Q14126	Desmoglein 2 preproprotein.	1.00	4	11		2	2
IPI00031620	P32942	Intercellular adhesion molecule 3.	1.00	17	71	CD50	2	1
IPI00072743	Q9NY35	Isoform 1 of claudin domain-containing protein 1.	1.00	2	10		4	4
IPI00107831	P10586	Receptor-type tyrosine-protein phosphatase F.	1.00	3	6		2	1
IPI00152540	Q6YHK3	Isoform 1 of CD109 antigen.	1.00	5	13	CD109	2	0
IPI00155168	P08575	Protein tyrosine phosphatase, receptor type, C.	1.00	9	42	CD45	2	2
IPI00157687	P16284	Isoform delta15 of platelet endothelial cell adhesion mol.	1.00	2	7	CD31	2	1
IPI00168812	Q8NFA6	Ptk7 protein tyrosine kinase 7 isoform D.	1.00	6	32		2	2
IPI00216514	Q08722	Isoform oa3-293 of leukocyte surface antigen CD47.	1.00	4	20	CD47	6	6
IPI00217561	P05556	Isoform beta-1c of integrin beta-1.	1.00	2	4	CD29	2	1
IPI00218795	P14151	L-selectin.	1.00	2	6	CD62L	1	1
IPI00220194	P11166	Solute carrier family 2, facilitated glucose transporter.	1.00	2	10		12	12
IPI00221240	Q9UIQ6	Isoform 2 of leucyl-cystinyl aminopeptidase.	1.00	3	10		1	1
IPI00291792	P05107	Integrin beta-2.	1.00	9	46	CD18	2	1
IPI00293074	Q8IWA5	Isoform 2 of choline transporter-like protein 2.	1.00	3	14		11	11
IPI00298702	Q13433	Isoform 1 of zinc transporter SLC39A6.	1.00	2	9		6	6
IPI00303401	Q6IA87	Uncharacterized protein C1ORF75.	1.00	2	8		2	1
IPI00306604	P08648	Integrin alpha-5.	1.00	5	14	CD49e	2	1
IPI00396658	Q9H0X4	Isoform 2 of protein ITFG3.	1.00	8	24		1	1
IPI00410600	Q9Y268	Calcium channel, voltage-dependent, alpha 2/delta.	1.00	3	5		0	0
IPI00431528	Q2YD82	TRA@ protein.	1.00	4	24		0	1
IPI00435872	O76082	Isoform 2 of organic cation/carnitine transporter 2.	1.00	3	6		11	12
IPI00445668	Q6ZUK4	Isoform 1 of transmembrane protein 26.	1.00	4	13		7	5
IPI00471951	Q07000	Hla class i histocompatibility antigen, CW-15 alpha.	1.00	2	9		2	1
IPI00550382	Q99808	Equilibrative nucleoside transporter 1.	1.00	2	10		11	11
IPI00552671	Q9UIW2	Plexin-A1.	1.00	2	10		2	2
IPI00783573	Q17RW0	Insulin receptor isoform short.	1.00	2	23	CD220	2	2
IPI00008494	P05362	Intercellular adhesion molecule 1.	1.00	2	7	CD54	2	1
IPI00018860	Q9BZM5	NNKGD ligand 2.	1.00	2	7		2	1
IPI00006644	O43157	Isoform 2 of plexin-B1.	1.00	2	5		2	0
IPI00004657	P01889	Hla class i histocompatibility antigen, B-7 alpha chain.	1.00	1	2		2	1
IPI00807403	Q13740	Isoform 2 of CD166 antigen.	1.00	2	5	CD166	2	1
IPI00013303	Q13449	Limbic system-associated membrane protein.	1.00	2	11		2	1

Supplemental Material

IPI ID	UniProt AC	Protein Name	PP	num unique peps	tot num peps	CD	Sosui TM	TM HMM
IPI00030431	Q9H6X2	Isoform 1 of anthrax toxin receptor 1.	1.00	2	7		2	1
IPI00176427	Q6NUR8	Immunoglobulin superfamily member 4c.	1.00	2	5		2	1
IPI00398435	O15031	Similar to plexin-B2.	1.00	2	5		3	0
IPI00013897	O14672	Adam 10.	1.00	2	4	CD156	2	1
IPI00015102	Q13740	Isoform 1 of CD166 antigen.	1.00	2	8	CD166	2	1
IPI00000795	Q63HQ0	Isoform 1 of uncharacterized protein C4ORF16.	1.00	1	1		0	0
IPI00009456	P21589	5'-Nucleotidase.	1.00	1	3	CD73	2	2
IPI00013435	P15813	T-cell surface glycoprotein CD1d.	1.00	1	1	CD1d	2	1
IPI00015756	Q15262	Receptor-type tyrosine-protein phosphatase kappa.	1.00	1	5		2	2
IPI00018901	P19440	Isoform 1 of gamma-glutamyltranspeptidase 1.	1.00	1	2	CD224	2	3
IPI00019472	Q15758	Neutral amino acid transporter b.	1.00	1	6		10	9
IPI00020446	P27701	Cd82 antigen.	1.00	1	1	CD82	4	4
IPI00021983	Q92542	Isoform 1 of nicastrin.	1.00	1	2		0	1
IPI00027281	P14672	Solute carrier family 2, facilitated glucose transporter.	1.00	1	1		11	12
IPI00030847	Q9HD45	Transmembrane 9 superfamily protein member 3.	1.00	1	2		9	9
IPI00289831	Q13332	Ptps of receptor-type tyrosine-protein phosphatase s.	1.00	1	2		2	2
IPI00299412	P48960	Isoform 2 of CD97 antigen.	1.00	1	5	CD97	8	7
IPI00329027	Q86VZ1	P2y purinoceptor 8.	1.00	1	2		8	6
IPI00394808	Q6PCB8	Embigin.	1.00	1	7		1	1
IPI00216985	P20023	Isoform b of complement receptor type 2.	0.99	1	4	CD21	2	1
IPI00289204	Q9BZR6	Reticulon-4 receptor.	0.99	1	13		0	0
IPI00419724	Q9NPR2	Semaphorin 4b.	0.99	1	5		2	1
IPI00032061	Q9P1W8	Isoform 1 of signal-regulatory protein gamma.	0.99	1	7	CD172	2	1
IPI00022284	P04156	Major prion protein.	0.99	1	6	CD230	2	2
IPI00398918	Q68D85	Hypothetical protein dkfzp686i21167.	0.99	1	2		3	2
IPI00006093	Q0KKZ9	Mib.	0.98	1	4		25	25
IPI00029756	Q12866	Proto-oncogene tyrosine-protein kinase mer.	0.98	1	1		2	1
IPI00016890	NA	Similar to immunoglobulin superfamily, member 3.	0.98	1	1		2	1
IPI00472202	P56199	Integrin alpha-1.	0.98	1	1	CD49a	3	1
IPI00215995	P26006	Isoform alpha-3a of integrin alpha-3.	0.98	1	1	CD49c	2	2
IPI00106689	Q8NBN3	Isoform 2 of transmembrane protein 87a.	0.98	1	3		1	0
IPI00008148	P56159	Isoform 1 of gdnf family receptor alpha-1.	0.97	1	4		1	0
IPI00010338	P13726	Tissue factor.	0.97	1	2	CD142	2	1
IPI00152377	Q8TCJ2	Dolichyl-diphosphooligosaccharide-protein.	0.97	1	2		11	10
IPI00003986	P01733	T-cell receptor beta chain v region yt35.	0.97	1	8		0	0
IPI00030687	Q06418	Tyrosine-protein kinase receptor tyro3.	0.96	1	3		3	1
IPI00025257	O75326	Semaphorin-7a.	0.96	1	2	CD108	0	0
IPI00013744	P17301	Integrin alpha-2.	0.96	1	3	CD49b	2	1
IPI00022558	O95297	Isoform 1 of myelin protein zero-like protein 1.	0.96	1	8		2	2
IPI00184019	Q9UKJ1	Isoform 2 of paired immunoglobulin-like type 2 receptor.	0.95	1	4		0	0
IPI00217882	Q99523	Sortilin.	0.93	1	3		2	1
IPI00022339	O14747	Isoform 1 of t-cell-specific surface glycoprotein CD28.	0.92	1	8	CD28	1	1
IPI00296869	P25116	Proteinase-activated receptor 1.	0.92	1	3		8	7
IPI00021275	P29323	Isoform 1 of ephrin type-b receptor 2.	0.91	1	5		2	1
IPI00375879	Q49AF2	Hypothetical protein loc57613.	0.91	1	4		2	1

Supplemental Material

Supplementary Table S3.2. CSC identified mouse splenocyte proteins. MS identified proteins from mouse splenocytes by using the CSC technology. Shown is the list of 87 protein identifications, including 36 CD proteins, with a ProteinProphet probability of 0.9 or higher. The specificity for CSC proteins is 93% The proteins were identified from one experimental sample which was run back to back two times under the same conditions on an LTQ-FT. The sample was run twice for statistical purposes in order to increase the confidence in the peptide identifications. Displayed columns include the IPI ID (Human V3.26); UniProt AC; Protein name; ProteinProphet probability (PP); the number of uniquely identified peptides/protein; the total number of identified peptides/protein; CD annotation; SOSUI and TMHMM transmembrane prediction.

IPI ID	UniProt AC	Protein Name	PP	num unique peps	tot num peps	CD	Sosui TM	TM HMM
IPI00109946	P18181	CD48 antigen.	1.00	3	6	CD48	2	0
IPI00113869	P18572	Isoform 2 of basigin.	1.00	3	8	CD147	2	1
IPI00115762	P11627	Neural cell adhesion molecule l1.	1.00	4	9	CD171	2	1
IPI00115892	P04441	H-2 class ii histocompatibility antigen gamma chain.	1.00	2	4	CD74	1	1
IPI00117140	Q5U677	Fcgr2b protein.	1.00	3	24		1	1
IPI00117424	P35330	Intercellular adhesion molecule 2.	1.00	5	9	CD102	2	1
IPI00118020	Q99N28	Immunoglobulin superfamily member 4b.	1.00	2	2		2	1
IPI00119063	Q91ZX7	Low-density lipoprotein receptor-related protein 1.	1.00	5	10		2	1
IPI00120674	Q3U1U4	B6-derived CD11 +ve dendritic cells cdna.	1.00	3	5		3	0
IPI00121334	Q00651	Integrin alpha-4.	1.00	4	5	CD49d	2	1
IPI00122257	Q61503	5'-Nucleotidase.	1.00	3	6	CD73	2	1
IPI00122973	Q9Z0M6	Isoform 1 of CD97 antigen.	1.00	4	7	CD97	8	7
IPI00124221	P97370	Sodium/potassium-transporting atpase subunit beta-3.	1.00	2	4	CD298	1	1
IPI00124830	Q61735	Isoform 2 of leukocyte surface antigen CD47.	1.00	5	11	CD47	6	5
IPI00126092	P06800	Isoform 2 of leukocyte common antigen.	1.00	5	11	CD45	2	2
IPI00129253	Q60767	Lymphocyte antigen 75.	1.00	3	6	CD205	2	1
IPI00129646	Q01965	T-lymphocyte surface antigen LY-9.	1.00	3	5	CD229	3	1
IPI00129968	P21995	Embigin.	1.00	6	12		2	1
IPI00130271	Q9Z1M0	P2x purinoceptor 7.	1.00	4	7		2	0
IPI00132286	P24063	Integrin alpha-l.	1.00	3	8	CD11a	2	1
IPI00169896	Q8BY89	Isoform 2 of choline transporter-like protein 2.	1.00	4	7		10	10
IPI00177214	Q8VCX7	Igh-6 protein.	1.00	5	10		2	1
IPI00223987	Q8C129	Leucyl-cystinyl aminopeptidase.	1.00	2	4		2	1
IPI00230289	P43006	Isoform 1a of excitatory amino acid transporter 2.	1.00	5	12		10	9
IPI00272690	P09470	Angiotensin-converting enzyme, somatic isoform.	1.00	2	3		2	1
IPI00405742	Q3UH76	Plexin b2.	1.00	4	7		3	0
IPI00406609	Q64455	Protein tyrosine phosphatase receptor type J.	1.00	8	15		1	1
IPI00406901	A2A6L8	Platelet/endothelial cell adhesion molecule.	1.00	4	6		2	1
IPI00463492	Q3UE15	Transmembrane protein 2.	1.00	2	3		1	1
IPI00785236	Q3T9T5	CD22 antigen.	1.00	4	9	CD22	2	1
IPI00110807	P01902	H-2 class I histocompatibility antigen, k-d alpha chain.	1.00	3	7		2	1
IPI00122973	P13597	Isoform 1 of intercellular adhesion molecule 1.	1.00	2	7	CD54	2	1
IPI00265854	P19070	Complement receptor type 2.	1.00	3	4	CD21	1	1
IPI00331175	Q9WVL3	Solute carrier family 12 member 7.	1.00	2	4		11	11
IPI00114274	O09126	Semaphorin-4d.	1.00	2	4	CD100	2	1
IPI00123831	P97300	Isoform 1 of neuroplastin.	1.00	3	5		2	1
IPI00322447	Q8K3T6	Immunoglobulin superfamily, member 4a isoform a.	1.00	2	3		2	1
IPI00396840	Q4PZA2	Isoform b of endothelin-converting enzyme 1.	1.00	2	3		2	1
IPI00109254	Q9EP73	Programmed cell death 1 ligand 1.	1.00	2	5	CD274	2	1
IPI00379131	Q3V0T4	Integrin alpha-d.	1.00	4	6	CD11d	1	1
IPI00108594	P01731	T-cell surface glycoprotein CD8 alpha chain.	1.00	3	10	CD8a	2	1
IPI00121740	P20693	Low affinity immunoglobulin epsilon fc receptor.	1.00	2	4	CD23	1	1
IPI00114256	O09117	Isoform 1 of synaptophysin-like protein 1.	1.00	1	2		4	3
IPI00119181	Q60677	Integrin alpha-e.	1.00	1	2		2	1
IPI00122522	Q60928	Gamma-glutamyltranspeptidase 1.	1.00	1	2	CD103	1	1
IPI00269413	Q2YFS3	Paired immunoglobulin-like type 2 receptor alpha.	1.00	1	2	CD224	1	1
IPI00314355	P21855	B-cell differentiation antigen CD72.	1.00	1	2	CD72	1	1
IPI00469000	Q8C145	Zinc transporter slc39a6.	1.00	1	2		6	6
IPI00785534	Q61895	Mrna. Precursor.	1.00	4	9		2	1
IPI00135324	P55012	Solute carrier family 12 member 2.	1.00	2	4		11	12
IPI00338209	Q9Z2A9	Isoform 1 of gamma-glutamyltransferase 5.	1.00	3	4		1	1
IPI00465769	Q91V14	Solute carrier family 12 member 5.	0.99	2	4		12	12
IPI00607925	Q9TQL9	Mhc class i antigen qa1 (fragment).	0.99	2	5		0	0
IPI00463120	Q61642	H-2k-sm1.	0.98	3	12		2	1
IPI00177200	P59222	Scavenger receptor class f member 2.	0.98	1	1		2	1
IPI00127869	Q9R100	Cadherin-17.	0.96	1	1		1	1
IPI00343568	Q62192	CD180 antigen.	0.96	1	2	CD180	2	1
IPI00126344	P14431	H-2 class i histocompatibility antigen, q9 alpha chain.	0.96	1	20		1	0
IPI00129158	P97797	Tyrosine-prot. phosphatase non-receptor type subst.	0.96	2	2	CD172	2	1

Supplemental Material

IPI ID	UniProt AC	Protein Name	PP	num unique peps	tot num peps	CD	Sosui TM	TM HMM
IPI00129594	Q18PI6	Isoform 1 of slam family member 5.	0.96	1	1	CD84	1	1
IPI00122368	Q9JJX6	Isoform c of p2x purinoceptor 4.	0.96	1	2		0	2
IPI00115038	O55001	Killer cell inhibitory receptor-like protein p91b.	0.96	1	1		2	1
IPI00117451	O70394	Interleukin-27 receptor subunit alpha.	0.95	1	2		0	0
IPI00263302	Q2TB02	cDNA sequence ay078069.	0.95	1	2		0	0
IPI00119809	O35649	Mama protein.	0.95	1	2		0	0
IPI00120793	P04925	Major prion protein.	0.94	1	1	CD230	2	2
IPI00320605	P11835	Integrin beta-2.	0.94	1	4	CD18	2	1
IPI00124785	Q9WUL5	Programmed cell death 1 ligand 2.	0.94	1	2	CD273	2	1
IPI00124987	Q00941	Granulocyte-macrophage colony-stim. factor receptor.	0.94	1	2	CD116	2	1
IPI00131495	Q8CJ91	Isoform 2 of CD209 antigen-like protein b.	0.94	1	2	CD209	0	0
IPI00118168	Q2VLH6	Scavenger receptor cysteine-rich type 1 protein m130.	0.93	1	1	CD163	2	2
IPI00128859	P06802	Ectonucleotide pyrophosphatase/phosphodiesterase.	0.93	2	3	CD203	1	1
IPI00121362	Q8VC39	F11 receptor.	0.93	1	2		2	1
IPI00114509	P04235	T-cell surface glycoprotein CD3 delta chain.	0.92	1	1	CD3d	2	1
IPI00411060	Q7TS39	Olfactory receptor olfr199.	0.92	1	1		6	6
IPI00129365	Q8VIH9	Urotensin ii receptor.	0.92	1	1		6	7
IPI00223178	Q3UP23	Transmembrane protein 26.	0.92	1	1		7	5
IPI00110508	P26011	Integrin beta-7.	0.91	1	4		2	1
IPI00114338	O08523	Isoform 1 of alpha-tectorin.	0.91	1	2		0	0
IPI00471423	Q9DBR4	Amyloid beta a4 precursor protein-binding family.	0.91	1	1		0	0
IPI00320420	Q06890	Clusterin.	0.90	1	2		1	0

Supplementary Table S3.3 CSC identified and quantified human Ramos and Jurkat lymphocyte proteins. MS identified proteins from Jurkat T and Ramos B lymphocytes by using the CSC technology. Shown is the list of 96 protein identifications, including 40 CD proteins, with a ProteinProphet probability of 0.9 or higher. The specificity for CSC proteins is 97%. The proteins were identified from one experimental sample which was run back to back three times under the same conditions on an LCQ-DecaXP. The sample was run three times for statistical purposes in order to increase the confidence in the peptide identifications. Displayed columns include the IPI ID (Human V3.26); UniProt AC; Protein name; ProteinProphet probability (PP); the number of uniquely identified peptides/protein; the total number of identified peptides/protein; CD annotation; SOSUI and TMHMM transmembrane prediction; XPRESS quantitation ratio mean and standard deviation (SD).

IPI ID	UniProt AC	Protein Name	PP	num unique peps	tot num peps	CD	Sosui TM	TM HMM	XPRESS ratio mean	SD
IPI00028015	Q6GTX8	Leukocyte-associated Ig-like receptor.	1.00	2	5	CD305	2	1	0.09	0.03
IPI00471951	Q07000	Hla class I histocompatibility antigen.	1.00	2	6		2	1	0.10	0.02
IPI00022368	Q14126	Desmoglein 2 preproprotein.	0.99	1	2		2	2	0.10	0.02
IPI00020446	P27701	CD82 antigen.	1.00	2	5	CD82	4	4	0.13	0.03
IPI00306604	P08648	Integrin alpha-5.	1.00	2	6	CD49e	2	1	0.14	0.02
IPI00031620	P32942	Intercellular adhesion molecule 3.	1.00	12	59	CD50	2	1	0.16	0.03
IPI00009803	P13612	Integrin alpha-4.	1.00	4	6	CD49d	2	1	0.18	0.03
IPI00014854	Q07108	Early activation antigen CD69.	0.99	1	3	CD69	1	1	0.18	0.05
IPI00217447	P22001	Potassium voltage-gated channel,.	0.99	1	3		5	5	0.20	0.02
IPI00152540	Q6YHK3	Isoform 1 of CD109 antigen.	1.00	4	10	CD109	2	0	0.21	0.05
IPI00337612	Q8N8Z6	Discoidin.	0.99	1	2		2	1	0.21	0.00
IPI00015091	P09564	T-cell antigen CD7.	1.00	2	5	CD7	2	1	0.22	0.03
IPI00022892	P04216	Thy-1 membrane glycoprotein.	1.00	2	4	CD90	2	1	0.22	0.02
IPI00026241	Q10589	Bone marrow stromal antigen 2.	1.00	3	7	CD317	2	2	0.22	0.10
IPI00298851	P48509	CD151 antigen.	0.99	1	2	CD151	3	4	0.22	0.00
IPI00008148	P56159	GDNF family receptor alpha-1.	1.00	2	4		1	0	0.24	0.01
IPI00013411	P15813	T-cell surface glycoprotein CD1d.	1.00	2	6	CD1d	2	1	0.24	0.05
IPI00552671	Q9UIW2	Plexin-a1.	0.99	1	3		2	2	0.24	0.03
IPI00031411	Q14517	Cadherin-related tumor suppressor.	1.00	2	4		2	1	0.27	0.07
IPI00021058	Q9Y6M7	Sodium bicarbonate cotransporter 3.	1.00	3	5		11	11	0.28	0.04
IPI00002236	Q08431	Lactadherin.	0.99	1	1		0	0	0.28	0.03
IPI00022039	Q9UIB8	Isoform 3 of slam family member 5.	0.99	1	3	CD84	2	1	0.31	0.01
IPI00023814	Q92859	Isoform 1 of neogenin.	1.00	4	10		2	1	0.32	0.07
IPI00015726	Q15262	Receptor-type tyr-protein phosphatase.	1.00	3	6		2	2	0.34	0.05
IPI00107831	P10586	Receptor-type tyr-protein phosphatase.	1.00	2	4		2	1	0.34	0.09
IPI00019850	P29017	T-cell surface glycoprotein CD1c.	0.99	1	3	CD1c	2	1	0.34	0.05
IPI00018860	Q9BZM5	Nkg2d ligand 2.	0.93	1	3		2	1	0.38	0.16

Supplemental Material

IPI ID	UniProt AC	Protein Name	PP	num unique peps	tot num peps	CD	Sosui TM	TM HMM	Xpress ratio mean	SD
IPI00008085	Q3MJA4	Solute carrier family 39.	1.00	4	7		8	7	0.39	0.08
IPI00023807	Q92854	Semaphorin-4d.	1.00	7	18	CD100	2	2	0.39	0.05
IPI00103356	Q8WWJ8	Integrin-like protein.	0.99	1	2		2	1	0.40	0.03
IPI00168812	Q8NFA6	Ptk7 protein tyrosine kinase 7.	0.99	1	2		2	2	0.40	0.00
IPI00016890	NA	Similar to Ig superfamily.	1.00	2	3		2	1	0.41	0.07
IPI00013744	P17301	Integrin alpha-2.	0.99	1	2	CD49b	2	1	0.43	0.10
IPI00027484	P06729	T-cell surface antigen CD2.	1.00	2	4	CD2	2	1	0.44	0.03
IPI00155168	P08575	Protein tyrosine phosphatase receptor.	1.00	10	30	CD45	2	1	0.44	0.04
IPI00221240	Q9UIQ6	Leucyl-cystinyl aminopeptidase.	1.00	2	6		1	1	0.44	0.02
IPI00219172	P29320	Isoform 2 of ephrin type-a receptor 3.	1.00	2	3		0	0	0.47	0.05
IPI00298702	Q13433	Isoform 1 of zinc transporter slc39a6.	1.00	2	4		6	6	0.47	0.01
IPI00303401	Q6IA87	Uncharacterized protein c1orf75.	1.00	2	6		2	1	0.47	0.04
IPI00005125	P52798	Isoform 1 of ephrin-a4.	0.99	1	1		2	0	0.48	0.00
IPI00216514	Q08722	Leukocyte surface antigen CD47.	0.93	3	4	CD47	6	6	0.50	0.10
IPI00030431	Q9H6X2	Isoform 1 of anthrax toxin receptor 1.	0.99	1	1		1	1	0.52	0.04
IPI00022558	O95297	Myelin protein zero-like protein 1.	0.96	1	1		2	2	0.55	0.00
IPI00015102	Q13740	Isoform 1 of CD166 antigen.	1.00	3	13	CD166	2	1	0.56	0.05
IPI00394808	Q6PCB8	Embigin.	1.00	6	16		1	1	0.57	0.19
IPI00003813	A0A4Z1	Nectin-like protein 2.	1.00	11	29		2	1	0.59	0.10
IPI00027728	P30825	High-affinity cationic AA transporter 1.	1.00	4	12		14	14	0.59	0.10
IPI00022462	P02786	Transferrin receptor protein 1.	1.00	8	17	CD71	1	1	0.64	0.06
IPI00024307	P98172	Ephrin-b1.	1.00	2	2		2	1	0.65	0.15
IPI00019906	P35613	Isoform 2 of basigin.	1.00	4	8	CD147	2	2	0.69	0.11
IPI00022649	P55011	Solute carrier family 12 member 2.	0.92	1	3		11	12	0.71	0.15
IPI00218795	P14151	L-selectin.	1.00	2	4	CD62L	1	1	0.76	0.30
IPI00644025	Q7L0J3	Synaptic vesicle glycoprotein 2a.	0.99	1	3		11	12	0.76	0.05
IPI00015476	P43007	Neutral amino acid transporter a.	1.00	4	9		9	9	0.80	0.33
IPI00396658	Q9H0X4	Isoform 2 of protein itfg3.	1.00	4	9		1	1	0.81	0.41
IPI00027281	P14672	Glucose transporter member 4.	0.99	2	2		11	12	0.81	0.00
IPI00012877	P17181	Interferon-alpha/beta receptor alpha.	1.00	2	5		2	2	0.82	0.07
IPI00099863	Q9NQ25	Isoform 1 of slam family member 7.	0.95	1	2	CD319	2	1	0.83	0.01
IPI00010193	P48551	Interferon-alpha/beta receptor beta.	0.99	1	1		1	1	0.85	0.00
IPI00021983	Q92542	Isoform 1 of nicastrin.	1.00	3	3		0	1	0.87	0.07
IPI00550382	Q99808	Equilibrative nucleoside transporter 1.	1.00	6	13		11	11	0.97	0.11
IPI00444383	P24394	Interleukin-4 receptor alpha chain.	0.98	1	3	CD124	2	0	0.98	0.09
IPI00397229	P48960	Isoform 1 of CD97 antigen.	1.00	3	6	CD97	8	7	0.99	0.21
IPI00003648	Q15223	Poliovirus receptor-related protein 1.	1.00	2	6	CD111	2	2	1.05	0.05
IPI00293074	Q8IWA5	Choline transporter-like protein 2.	1.00	3	5	CD211	11	11	1.10	0.10
IPI00027232	P08069	Insulin-like growth factor 1 receptor.	1.00	2	5	CD221	2	1	1.17	0.07
IPI00025803	P06213	Insulin receptor.	1.00	2	4	CD220	2	2	1.24	0.13
IPI00220194	P11166	Glucose transporter member 1.	1.00	4	13		12	12	1.31	0.17
IPI00385059	Q7Z3Y6	Rearranged vh4-34 v gene segment.	1.00	2	2		0	0	1.32	0.12
IPI00002478	P42892	Endothelin-converting enzyme 1.	1.00	7	14		1	1	1.51	0.35
IPI00018282	P25942	Isoform I of TNF receptor superfamily.	0.99	1	2	CD40	2	1	1.60	0.23
IPI00064951	Q96LA6	Fc receptor-like protein 1.	0.97	1	1		0	1	1.68	0.00
IPI00027459	P08195	4F2 cell-surface antigen heavy chain.	1.00	24	139	CD98	1	1	1.73	0.54
IPI00171334	Q9H015	Organic cation/carnitine transporter 1.	0.99	1	2		12	11	1.75	0.03
IPI00008473	P11912	B-cell antigen receptor complex.	1.00	3	7	CD79a	2	1	1.80	0.38
IPI00513714	Q5TAS6	Slam family member 6.	0.98	1	1		2	1	1.86	0.00
IPI00177968	Q8WTV0	Scavenger receptor class b member 1.	0.99	1	2		3	2	2.44	0.12
IPI00219131	O75144	Isoform 1 of icos ligand.	1.00	2	6	CD275	1	1	2.45	0.41
IPI00148599	Q96M80	Cell recognition protein CASPR4.	0.98	1	1		0	0	2.49	0.00
IPI00218390	P20273	CD22-alpha of b-cell receptor CD22.	0.99	1	3	CD22	3	1	3.07	0.97
IPI00029606	P78536	Isoform b of adam 17.	0.92	1	1	CD156	2	1	3.21	0.00
IPI00152871	Q8TF66	Leucine-rich repeat-containing protein.	0.96	1	2		1	1	3.41	0.23
IPI00398435	O15031	Similar to plexin-b2.	1.00	8	22		3	0	3.79	1.63
IPI00003400	P11049	Leukocyte antigen CD37.	0.99	1	5	CD37	3	4	4.04	1.55
IPI00021711	P20036	Hla class ii histocompatibility antigen.	1.00	1	6		1	1	4.24	0.74
IPI00015696	Q5T2D2	Receptor expressed on myeloid cells.	0.98	1	1		1	1	4.38	0.00
IPI00001922	Q9Y5Y6	Suppressor of tumorigenicity protein.	1.00	2	28		1	1	4.45	2.62
IPI00175654	A1L458	Similar to mast cell antigen 32.	0.99	1	1		1	1	4.62	0.78
IPI00027381	O60449	Isoform 1 of lymphocyte antigen 75.	1.00	3	7	CD205	2	1	5.15	1.76
IPI00008494	P05362	Intercellular adhesion molecule 1.	1.00	5	12	CD54	1	1	5.32	0.82
IPI00006071	P28907	Isoform 1 of adp-ribosyl cyclase 1.	1.00	6	15	CD38	1	1	5.92	1.93
IPI00027668	P40259	B-cell antigen receptor complex.	1.00	3	9	CD79b	2	1	15.65	5.03
IPI00005171	P01903	Hla class II histocompatibility antigen.	1.00	4	12		2	1	17.94	6.43

Supplemental Material

Supplementary Table S3.4 CSC identified and quantified proteins from unstimulated and CD3/CD28 stimulated human Jurkat T lymphopcytes. MS identified proteins from unstimulated and CD3/CD28 stimulated Jurkat T lymphocytes by using the CSC technology. Shown is the list of 119 protein identifications, includig 47 CD proteins, with a ProteinProphet probability of 0.9 or higher. The specificity for CSC proteins is 94%. The proteins were identified from one experimental sample which was run back to back four times under the same conditions on an LTQ-FT. The sample was run four times for statistical purposes in order to increase the confidence in the peptide identifications and quantification. Displayed columns include the IPI ID (Human v3.26); UniProt AC; Protein name; ProteinProphet probability (PP); the number of uniquely identified peptides/protein; the total number of identified peptides/protein; CD annotation; SOSUI and TMHMM transmembrane prediction; XPRESS quantitation ratio mean normalized.

IPI ID	UniProt AC	Protein Name	PP	num unique peps	tot num peps	CD	Sosui TM	TM HMM	XPRESS ratio mean normalized
IPI00184311	P22413	Ectonucleotide pyrophosphatase.	1.00	6	14		1	1	0.04
IPI00014854	Q07108	Early activation antigen CD69.	1.00	6	21	CD69	1	1	0.07
IPI00106689	Q8NBN3	Isoform 2 of transmembrane protein 87a.	1.00	2	2		1	0	0.29
IPI00289819	P11717	Cation-indep. man-6-phosphate receptor.	0.97	2	7	CD222	3	1	0.34
IPI00000877	Q9Y4L1	150 Kda oxygen-regulated protein.	0.94	2	3		1	1	0.36
IPI00553238	Q69YH1	CDna flj42617 fis, clone brace3014807.	0.98	1	1		5	3	0.39
IPI00013303	Q13449	Limbic system-assoc. membrane protein.	1.00	4	11		2	1	0.46
IPI00013744	P17301	Integrin alpha-2.	1.00	2	3	CD49b	2	1	0.46
IPI00009456	P21589	5'-Nucleotidase.	1.00	2	3	CD73	2	2	0.46
IPI00020446	P27701	CD82 antigen.	1.00	4	6	CD82	4	4	0.51
IPI00397229	P48960	Isoform 1 of CD97 antigen.	1.00	9	13	CD97	8	7	0.58
IPI00155168	P08575	Protein tyrosine phosphatase receptor.	1.00	36	147	CD45	2	2	0.60
IPI00022284	P04156	Major prion protein.	1.00	2	12	CD230	2	2	0.60
IPI00184175	Q9BZW8	Isoform 2 of natural killer cell receptor 2b4.	0.98	2	3	CD244	2	1	0.60
IPI00023807	Q92854	Semaphorin-4d.	1.00	12	37	CD100	2	1	0.61
IPI00028931	Q14126	Desmoglein 2 preproprotein.	1.00	4	7		2	2	0.61
IPI00783166	NA	Similar to ribosomal protein l7-like 1.	1.00	2	6		2	1	0.61
IPI00006071	P28907	Isoform 1 of adp-ribosyl cyclase 1.	1.00	6	13	CD38	1	1	0.63
IPI00217892	Q99523	Sortilin.	1.00	6	15		2	1	0.63
IPI00445668	Q6ZUK4	Isoform 1 of transmembrane protein 26.	1.00	3	6		7	5	0.63
IPI00021275	P29323	Isoform 1 of ephrin type-b receptor 2.	1.00	2	3		2	1	0.64
IPI00293074	Q8IWA5	Choline transporter-like protein 2.	1.00	4	17		11	11	0.66
IPI00306604	P08648	Integrin alpha-5.	1.00	13	35	CD49e	2	1	0.68
IPI00183782	NA	72 Kda protein.	1.00	3	9	CD229	2	1	0.68
IPI00027604	P40200	T-cell surface protein tactile.	1.00	9	29	CD96	2	1	0.70
IPI00152540	Q9YHK3	Isoform 1 of CD109 antigen.	1.00	2	2	CD109	2	0	0.70
IPI00303401	Q6IA87	Uncharacterized protein c1orf75.	1.00	2	9		2	1	0.70
IPI00019472	Q15758	Neutral amino acid transporter b.	1.00	4	8		10	9	0.75
IPI00027493	P08195	4F2 cell-surface antigen heavy chain.	1.00	87	390	CD98	1	1	0.75
IPI00021058	Q9Y6M7	Sodium bicarbonate cotransporter 3.	1.00	9	18		11	11	0.75
IPI00015476	P43007	Neutral amino acid transporter a.	1.00	11	76		9	9	0.81
IPI00014236	Q15043	Solute carrier family 39 member 14.	1.00	11	20		4	6	0.81
IPI00396658	Q9H0X4	Isoform 2 of protein itfg3.	1.00	10	27		1	1	0.83
IPI00022558	O95297	Myelin protein zero-like protein 1.	1.00	3	17		2	1	0.83
IPI00221240	Q9UIQ6	Leucyl-cystinyl aminopeptidase.	1.00	22	61		1	1	0.83
IPI00298702	Q13433	Isoform 1 of zinc transporter slc39a6.	1.00	5	10		6	8	0.84
IPI00736324	Q5TAS4	Slam family member 6.	1.00	6	16		2	1	0.86
IPI00031411	O14517	Cadherin-related tumor suppressor.	1.00	3	4		2	1	0.87
IPI00002478	P42892	Endothelin-converting enzyme 1.	1.00	11	27		1	1	0.88
IPI00012977	O00478	Butyrophilin subfamily 3 member a3.	1.00	2	4		1	1	0.91
IPI00151710	Q4KMQ2	Transmembrane protein 16f.	1.00	2	11		8	7	0.91
IPI00298748	Q6PCB8	Embigin.	1.00	2	11		1	1	0.91
IPI00003813	A0A4Z1	Nectin-like protein 2.	1.00	9	29		2	1	0.93
IPI00008167	P54709	Na/K-transporting ATPase subunit beta-3.	1.00	5	28	CD298	2	1	0.93
IPI00009803	P13612	Integrin alpha-4.	1.00	22	62	CD49d	2	1	0.93
IPI00011578	Q9Y639	Isoform 1 of neuroplastin.	1.00	7	18		1	1	0.95
IPI00027728	P30825	High-affinity cationic AA transporter 1.	1.00	9	23		14	14	0.95
IPI00216514	Q08722	Leukocyte surface antigen CD47.	1.00	9	43	CD47	6	6	0.95
IPI00552671	Q9UIW2	Plexin-a1.	1.00	4	13		2	2	0.96
IPI00019850	P29017	T-cell surface glycoprotein CD1c.	1.00	9	16	CD1c	2	1	0.98
IPI00030431	Q9H6X2	Isoform 1 of anthrax toxin receptor 1.	1.00	2	8		2	1	0.98
IPI00168812	Q8NFA6	Ptk7 protein tyrosine kinase 7 isoform d.	1.00	21	59		2	1	0.98
IPI00291792	P05107	Integrin beta-2.	1.00	21	99	CD18	2	1	0.99

Supplemental Material

IPI ID	UniProt AC	Protein Name	PP	num unique peps	tot num peps	CD	Sosui TM	TM HMM	XPRESS ratio mean normalized
IPI00645194	Q8WUM6	Integrin beta 1 isoform 1a.	1.00	10	24	CD29	2	1	1.01
IPI00472162	Q29865	Hla class I histocompatibility antigen.	0.99	3	9		2	1	1.02
IPI00216985	P20023	Isoform b of complement receptor type 2.	1.00	2	7	CD21	2	1	1.06
IPI00783573	Q17RW0	Insulin receptor isoform short.	1.00	4	10	CD220	2	2	1.06
IPI00013831	P09326	CD48 antigen.	1.00	13	50	CD48	2	1	1.07
IPI00015756	Q15262	Receptor-type tyr-protein phosphatase k.	1.00	3	9		2	2	1.08
IPI00742977	NA	24 Kda protein.	0.99	4	12		1	0	1.10
IPI00022649	P55011	Solute carrier family 12 member 2.	1.00	2	3		11	12	1.10
IPI00027505	P06756	Integrin alpha-v.	1.00	2	6	CD51	2	1	1.10
IPI00747849	P05026	Na/K-transporting atpase subunit beta-1.	1.00	6	14		1	1	1.10
IPI00008494	P05362	Intercellular adhesion molecule 1.	1.00	6	15	CD54	2	1	1.11
IPI00019906	P35613	Isoform 2 of basigin.	1.00	16	67	CD147	2	2	1.12
IPI00332947	NA	31 Kda protein.	0.97	2	8		1	1	1.12
IPI00026241	Q10589	Bone marrow stromal antigen 2.	1.00	4	13	CD317	2	1	1.15
IPI00027281	P14672	Glucose transporter member 4.	1.00	2	3		11	12	1.15
IPI00107831	P10586	Receptor-type tyr-protein phosphatase f.	1.00	2	4		2	1	1.19
IPI00471951	Q07000	Hla class I histocompatibility antigen.	1.00	8	24		2	1	1.19
IPI00219172	P29320	Isoform 2 of ephrin type-a receptor 3.	0.94	1	2		0	0	1.20
IPI00018901	P19440	Gamma-glutamyltranspeptidase 1.	1.00	2	3	CD224	2	3	1.20
IPI00072743	Q9NY35	Claudin domain-containing protein 1.	1.00	3	9		4	4	1.21
IPI00022892	P04216	Thy-1 membrane glycoprotein.	1.00	13	47	CD90	2	0	1.22
IPI00012877	P17181	Interferon-alpha/beta receptor alpha chain.	1.00	4	5		2	2	1.24
IPI00031620	P32942	Intercellular adhesion molecule 3.	1.00	54	263	CD50	2	1	1.26
IPI00019381	Q9NV96	Isoform 1 of cell cycle control protein 50a.	1.00	8	18		2	2	1.30
IPI00011642	P23468	Receptor-type tyr-protein phosphatase d.	0.98	2	4		2	1	1.30
IPI00013435	O14672	T-cell surface glycoprotein CD1d.	1.00	3	9	CD1d	2	1	1.32
IPI00013897	O14672	Adam 10.	1.00	5	14	CD156	2	1	1.34
IPI00022339	P10747	T-cell-specific surface glycoprotein CD28.	1.00	6	23	CD28	1	1	1.34
IPI00032061	Q9P1W8	Signal-regulatory protein gamma.	1.00	2	11	CD172	2	1	1.34
IPI00023814	Q92859	Isoform 1 of neogenin.	1.00	9	21		2	1	1.37
IPI00022462	P02786	Transferrin receptor protein 1.	1.00	11	45	CD71	1	1	1.38
IPI00009477	P13598	Intercellular adhesion molecule 2.	1.00	34	134	CD102	2	1	1.38
IPI00019862	Q96AV7	Butyrophilin, subfamily 2, member a1.	1.00	2	6		2	2	1.42
IPI00220194	P11166	Glucose transporter member 1.	1.00	7	32		12	12	1.54
IPI00550382	Q99808	Equilibrative nucleoside transporter 1.	1.00	4	16		11	11	1.55
IPI00152850	Q9BX67	Junctional adhesion molecule 3.	1.00	2	3		1	1	1.57
IPI00003648	Q15223	Poliovirus receptor-related protein 1.	1.00	6	22	CD111	2	2	1.62
IPI00006093	Q0KKZ9	Mib.	1.00	2	5		25	25	1.64
IPI00157687	P16284	Platelet endothel. cell adhesion molecule.	1.00	5	8	CD31	2	1	1.65
IPI00025380	P20701	Isoform 1 of integrin alpha-l.	1.00	4	9	CD11a	2	2	1.71
IPI00028015	Q6GTX8	Leukocyte-associated IG-like receptor 1.	1.00	4	21	CD305	2	2	1.75
IPI00019849	P29016	Isoform 1 of t-cell surface glycoprotein.	1.00	4	9	CD1b	2	1	1.79
IPI00431528	Q2YD82	Tra@ protein.	1.00	8	38		0	1	1.85
IPI00216143	NA	70 Kda protein.	1.00	2	7		12	12	1.93
IPI00015199	P09564	T-cell antigen CD7.	1.00	8	27	CD7	2	1	1.98
IPI00006003	Q01151	CD83 antigen.	1.00	3	6	CD83	2	1	2.10
IPI00171334	Q9H015	Organic cation/carnitine transporter 1.	1.00	4	12		12	11	2.13
IPI00218795	P14151	L-selectin.	1.00	4	14	CD62L	1	1	2.18
IPI00166668	Q8N3Z8	Trbv21-1 protein.	0.99	3	19		0	0	2.20
IPI00003987	P01737	T-cell receptor alpha chain v region py14.	1.00	2	6		2	0	3.03
IPI00003986	P01733	T-cell receptor beta chain v region yt35.	1.00	2	11		0	0	3.08
IPI00374077	Q5JX69	Uncharacterized protein c20orf107.	1.00	2	5		2	2	3.08
IPI00018860	Q9BZM5	Nkg2d ligand 2.	1.00	4	6		2	1	3.17
IPI00105102	Q13740	Isoform 1 of CD166 antigen.	0.99	0	0	CD166	2	1	NA
IPI00748835	Q6ZS95	Highly similar to CD166 antigen.	0.98	0	0		1	1	NA
IPI00783803	NA	65 Kda protein.	0.98	0	0		2	1	NA
IPI00004657	P01889	Hla class I histocompatibility antigen.	0.99	4	16		2	1	NA
IPI00013414	Q9BSF9	Mgc13005 protein.	0.99	2	9		2	0	0.00

Supplemental Material

Supplementary Table S4.1 CSC atlas - MS identified proteins from *D. melanogaster* Kc167 cell line using the CSC technology. Shown is the list of 202 protein identifications with a ProteinProphet probability of 0.9 or higher. The proteins were identified from 12 experiments which were run altogether 90 LC-MS/MS runs analyzed on an LTQ-FT. The cell surface atlas consists of 202 unique glycoproteins. Displayed columns include the protein name, protein probability, percent coverage (COV), number of unique and total number of peptides identified; the number of transmembrane (TM) domain as predicted by SOSUI and TMHMM as well as the gene ontology annotation for cellular component.

Protein Name	PP	COV	num unique peps	tot num peps	Sosui TM	TM HMM	GO: cellular component
almondex (Q9U4H5)	1.00	12.0	2	7	2	2	NA
arrow (Q95V09)	1.00	1.6	2	8	3	1	membrane
Saposin-related (Q86PA4)	1.00	3.4	3	26	1	0	intracellular
Fasciclin 1 (P10674)	1.00	10.9	35	742	2	0	membrane
Fasciclin 2 (P34082)	1.00	5.2	3	15	2	1	membrane
halfway (Q9W568)	1.00	22.1	35	422	2	0	NA
inflated (P12080)	0.99	1.1	1	18	2	2	membrane
Gliotactin (Q7YU32)	0.97	1.9	1	3	2	2	membrane
Laminin A (Q00174)	1.00	3.6	8	35	1	0	extracellular matrix
Laminin B1 (P11046)	1.00	2.1	3	39	1	0	extracellular matrix
Neuroglian (P20241)	1.00	6.6	12	59	2	1	membrane
Papilin (Q868Z9)	1.00	1.9	3	13	0	0	extracellular matrix
Activin receptor (Q24229)	1.00	8.1	8	112	2	1	membrane
Integrin alpha-PS3 (O44386)	1.00	3.0	4	126	2	1	membrane
smoothened (P91682)	0.99	1.0	1	2	8	6	membrane
Suppressor of variegation 3-9 (Q24208)	0.99	1.7	1	10	0	0	intracellular
Tropomyosin 1 (P06754)	1.00	4.3	4	8	0	0	intracellular
unzipped (P10379)	1.00	2.7	4	125	1	1	membrane
Neurotactin (P23654)	1.00	5.2	5	70	1	1	membrane
Protein tyrosine phosphatase 4E (Q24495)	1.00	2.6	3	40	1	2	membrane
Protein tyrosine phosphatase 10D (P35992)	1.00	1.3	2	5	1	2	membrane
Tenascin major (O18366)	1.00	3.7	5	148	1	1	membrane
Integrin alpha-PS1 (Q24247)	1.00	12.0	27	332	2	1	membrane
Integrin beta-PS (P11584)	1.00	13.7	26	316	2	1	membrane
off-track (Q24327)	1.00	1.8	3	19	2	2	membrane
roundabout (O44924)	1.00	4.1	6	20	1	1	membrane
Lachesin (Q24372)	1.00	4.7	3	22	2	0	membrane
beta[nu] integrin (Q27591)	0.94	2.3	1	11	2	1	membrane
lethal (2) 08717 (Q8MRP7)	0.99	1.4	1	34	10	11	membrane
cueball (Q95RU0)	1.00	11.5	30	434	2	1	membrane
Basigin (Q8IPG9)	1.00	39.6	59	1753	2	1	NA
Sema-1a (Q24322)	1.00	5.5	2	3	2	2	membrane
Sema-2a (Q24323)	1.00	3.2	2	19	1	0	extracellular matrix
baboon (Q23975)	1.00	7.8	5	52	2	1	membrane
Oligosaccharyl transferase 3 (Q9XZ53)	1.00	2.5	9	42	13	13	membrane
division abnormally delayed (Q24114)	1.00	5.8	12	63	2	0	extracellular matrix
frazzled (Q94537)	1.00	6.4	13	169	2	2	membrane
Malvolio (P49283)	1.00	6.2	4	15	11	9	membrane
Peroxidasin (Q23991)	0.97	0.7	1	1	1	0	membrane
Gp150 (Q24007)	1.00	2.0	2	3	2	1	membrane
Guanylyl cyclase at 76C (Q24051)	1.00	6.6	13	213	2	0	membrane
Insulin receptor (P09208)	1.00	10.0	60	1437	2	0	membrane
Neurexin IV (Q94887)	1.00	4.7	9	26	2	1	membrane
Protein tyrosine phosphatase 69D (P16620)	1.00	7.6	26	308	1	1	membrane
kekkon-1 (P91643)	1.00	4.4	2	2	2	1	membrane
Calnexin 99A (O02393)	1.00	2.1	2	111	2	1	intracellular
nervana 1 (Q24046)	1.00	7.4	12	151	1	1	membrane
nervana 2 (Q24048)	1.00	3.4	3	46	1	1	membrane
kuzbanian (Q94902)	1.00	8.9	25	330	1	1	NA
Sema-1b (O44253)	1.00	5.1	2	7	2	2	membrane
Macroglobulin complement-related (Q9VLT3)	1.00	3.9	11	115	2	1	NA
Imaginal disc growth factor 1 (Q8MM24)	0.99	4.3	1	5	0	0	NA
sidekick (O97134)	0.99	0.4	1	3	2	1	NA
Tyrosine-protein kinase receptor torso (Q9VKX7)	1.00	3.6	2	5	1	0	NA
Chitinase 2 (Q9W092)	1.00	8.3	5	12	0	0	NA

Supplemental Material

Protein Name	PP	COV	num unique peps	tot num peps	Sosui TM	TM HMM	GO: cellular component
methuselah (O97148)	1.00	3.1	2	12	6	7	membrane
CG2918 (O46067)	0.99	1.4	1	3	2	0	NA
Niemann-Pick Type C-1 (Q7YU59)	1.00	8.3	24	592	12	14	membrane
CG5594 (Q8MKK5)	1.00	3.3	15	224	11	10	membrane
plexin B (Q9V4A7)	1.00	3.2	10	58	2	3	membrane
plexin A (O96681)	1.00	6.0	14	186	1	0	membrane
Eph receptor tyrosine kinase (O96435)	1.00	5.3	6	70	3	1	membrane
prominin-like (P82295)	1.00	3.3	6	73	7	6	membrane
Equilibrative nucleoside transporter 2 (Q9VMB6)	1.00	3.1	8	200	9	11	membrane
CG3638 (Q8IRY1)	1.00	3.3	2	22	6	4	NA
CG9634 (Q9XZ14)	0.99	1.1	1	4	1	1	membrane
lethal (1) G0289 (Q9W2V9)	1.00	5.8	4	8	2	1	membrane
capulet (Q9VPX7)	0.93	1.2	1	1	0	0	membrane
CG10221 (Q9V415)	0.98	1.0	1	4	1	1	membrane
CG31731 (Q960V4)	1.00	3.0	11	182	11	11	membrane
Nhe3 (Q8IPJ4)	0.99	2.2	1	10	10	12	membrane
methuselah-like 3 (Q9V818)	1.00	5.0	3	25	7	7	membrane
26-29kD-proteinase (Q9V3U6)	0.99	2.6	1	18	1	0	NA
dispatched (Q8SY40)	1.00	3.9	3	10	12	12	membrane
Tollo (Q9V477)	1.00	4.1	6	37	2	2	membrane
NtR (Q8T9A2)	1.00	5.0	2	3	5	4	membrane
Hemolectin (Q8MS79)	1.00	2.9	13	125	1	0	extracellular matrix
CG12688 (Q9W4K7)	0.92	6.7	1	1	0	0	NA
CG3033 (Q961V1)	0.97	2.4	1	1	6	5	membrane
CG15347 (Q9W3F3)	1.00	29.4	7	74	2	0	NA
CG10353 (Q8MT62)	1.00	4.4	11	101	6	9	NA
CG15744 (Q95RH1)	1.00	3.6	5	33	7	6	membrane
CG11655 (Q9VXV4)	0.99	4.0	1	13	8	9	membrane
CG9917 (Q95SC0)	1.00	17.9	5	41	1	1	NA
CG9947 (Q8STD2)	1.00	8.1	7	177	2	2	membrane
CG4829 (Q8T0R6)	1.00	7.9	14	184	1	1	NA
unpaired 2 (Q9VWX2)	0.98	2.5	2	5	1	0	NA
CG7453 (Q8IQX2)	0.98	5.3	1	2	2	1	NA
CG14225 (Q9VWE1)	1.00	11.9	21	364	2	0	NA
CG14235 (Q8IQW2)	0.98	10.4	1	8	0	0	intracellular
CG1518 (Q9VRE0)	1.00	2.2	6	20	12	12	membrane
CG1718 (Q9VRG4)	0.98	1.0	1	3	12	14	membrane
nicotinic acetylcholine receptor beta 21C (Q8IPV6)	1.00	11.3	8	319	5	3	membrane
CG2813 (Q9VPR7)	1.00	10.5	6	80	2	2	NA
CG3662 (Q8T0C2)	0.99	4.8	1	1	1	1	NA
CG4726 (Q9VCU3)	1.00	10.4	29	283	12	10	membrane
CG17660 (Q961L7)	0.99	4.1	1	26	9	7	membrane
interference Hedgehog (Q9VM64)	0.99	1.2	1	21	2	1	membrane
peste (Q8SXU4)	0.99	2.2	1	33	3	2	membrane
CG8486 (Q8IPG4)	1.00	2.1	12	215	32	38	NA
PDGF- and VEGF-receptor related (Q8IPG1)	1.00	10.1	61	582	1	1	membrane
CG31886 (Q8SX26)	1.00	2.5	2	18	2	1	NA
CG5708 (Q9VL21)	0.98	5.0	1	9	0	0	NA
CG4972 (Q9VM25)	1.00	3.4	5	59	2	1	NA
CG16974 (Q95S21)	0.99	1.3	1	10	2	0	membrane
CadN2 (Q9VJB6)	1.00	1.4	3	5	2	2	membrane
CG10702 (Q9VJ04)	0.99	1.2	1	5	3	1	membrane
CG16771 (Q9VIW9)	1.00	6.4	11	160	1	1	NA
CG2493 (Q9VIM0)	1.00	4.6	2	93	1	0	intracellular
CG9318 (Q9VIK1)	0.95	1.2	1	5	10	9	membrane
CG9248 (Q9VIF2)	1.00	5.7	2	5	0	0	membrane
CG9247 (Q8MSZ9)	0.99	3.5	2	2	0	0	intracellular
CG3305 (Q8SZP0)	1.00	19.8	12	113	2	2	membrane
gp210 (Q9GPI0)	0.99	0.6	1	14	2	1	membrane
SCAP (Q8MRU6)	0.97	1.7	2	6	7	7	membrane
CG3271 (Q9V9C0)	0.99	4.9	1	5	6	7	NA
Tetraspanin 42EI (Q9V4G9)	1.00	5.5	3	90	4	4	membrane
Cirl (Q8SZV1)	1.00	3.8	9	165	7	8	membrane
CG9027 (Q95T42)	1.00	20.4	9	66	1	0	NA
CG12370 (Q8ML21)	0.99	3.4	1	3	8	6	membrane
straightjacket (Q95R75)	1.00	4.0	6	35	1	1	membrane
CG8399 (Q8MSU3)	1.00	3.1	13	64	7	6	NA
Dystroglycan (Q86BD9)	1.00	11.7	9	31	2	2	NA

Supplemental Material

Protein Name	PP	COV	num unique peps	tot num peps	Sosui TM	TM HMM	GO: cellular component
lambik (Q95RL4)	1.00	4.8	5	88	1	2	membrane
CG4827 (Q9VPD3)	0.98	1.7	1	1	1	0	NA
CG12263 (Q7YU86)	1.00	4.2	2	4	15	14	NA
CG15073 (Q8SYU8)	0.96	4.0	2	4	0	0	intracellular
CG11961 (Q8IH56)	1.00	1.3	3	87	9	9	NA
CG10062 (Q9V8T9)	1.00	1.0	2	2	9	9	NA
CG10444 (Q8SWV5)	1.00	2.7	3	32	11	13	membrane
CG16868 (Q9V917)	0.92	0.7	1	1	2	1	membrane
CG9304 (Q8T056)	0.92	3.1	1	5	8	7	NA
Organic anion transporting polypeptide 58Dc (Q9W269)	1.00	11.8	27	295	7	12	membrane
CG3907 (Q6IDE2)	1.00	2.8	2	33	1	1	NA
CG2213 (Q9W0G6)	0.96	2.8	1	4	0	0	NA
CG9953 (Q8SZM1)	1.00	2.0	2	6	1	1	membrane
CG8560 (Q961J8)	1.00	4.1	2	11	1	0	NA
wntless (Q95ST2)	0.99	2.0	1	8	9	8	NA
CG6199 (Q8MSV4)	1.00	5.5	7	26	0	0	intracellular
Sug (Q86PB0)	1.00	3.1	2	7	9	11	membrane
CG6038 (Q9VTM6)	0.97	6.3	1	1	2	0	NA
Transferrin 2 (Q9VTZ5)	1.00	3.1	2	6	2	0	NA
CG17667 (Q9VU13)	1.00	14.4	12	160	2	1	NA
CG7739 (Q9VUQ7)	1.00	5.5	3	6	2	1	NA
CG5235 (Q9VG74)	1.00	9.0	5	22	2	0	NA
CG5284 (Q8IQN2)	1.00	1.6	2	14	10	11	membrane
Organic anion transporting polypeptide 74D (Q8SWY1)	1.00	3.7	5	21	8	12	membrane
Adenosine deaminase-related growth factor A (Q9VVK5)	1.00	5.2	4	37	0	0	extracellular matrix
CG3797 (P10083)	0.98	1.7	1	3	3	2	NA
fat2 (Q9VW71)	1.00	0.9	5	26	2	1	membrane
CG5976 (Q86PD7)	1.00	3.1	3	51	0	0	NA
CG3618 (Q9W130)	1.00	3.4	3	19	2	0	NA
CG1092 (Q8SZJ1)	0.99	3.5	1	3	1	2	NA
Contactin (Q9VN14)	1.00	10.4	30	374	1	0	membrane
CG2791 (Q8SYR7)	1.00	19.3	40	751	1	1	NA
CG7800 (Q95SP1)	1.00	21.2	40	792	0	0	NA
CG8507 (Q9VH64)	0.99	2.6	1	21	1	1	intracellular
Tetraspanin 86D (Q9VGV3)	1.00	4.5	9	106	4	4	membrane
CG14713 (Q9VGK5)	0.99	2.9	1	7	1	1	NA
Cad87A (Q9VGG5)	1.00	1.6	3	37	3	1	membrane
CG9796 (Q95RA9)	1.00	5.2	3	93	1	0	NA
CG14857 (Q9VFG0)	1.00	1.8	2	28	10	11	membrane
CG5399 (Q9W1M4)	1.00	23.9	5	14	2	0	NA
CG3303 (Q9VF14)	1.00	3.4	2	5	1	1	NA
CG6126 (Q961R9)	1.00	5.8	6	36	12	11	membrane
CG7702 (Q9VE49)	0.98	1.9	1	4	2	1	NA
CG5382 (Q9VKZ6)	1.00	7.4	2	5	1	1	intracellular
wolfram syndrome 1 (P23128)	0.99	1.2	1	1	11	9	NA
CG17119 (Q9VCR7)	0.99	2.8	1	21	6	7	membrane
CG5789 (Q9VC63)	1.00	4.4	5	96	11	11	membrane
nicastrin (Q9VC27)	1.00	13.4	14	95	0	1	membrane
CG13654 (Q9VBW1)	1.00	4.2	2	3	7	7	membrane
CG11851 (Q9VBV8)	1.00	4.0	3	15	8	9	NA
CG6490 (Q8T986)	1.00	4.2	6	33	1	1	membrane
distracted (Q960R8)	1.00	2.8	2	10	1	1	membrane
CG11880 (Q8MR01)	1.00	4.1	13	186	9	10	NA
CG14516 (Q8SYT3)	1.00	1.8	5	54	1	1	NA
prolyl-4-hydroxylase-alpha EFB (Q9VA269)	1.00	5.8	2	21	1	1	NA
CG2126 (Q8SXK7)	0.99	3.6	1	1	6	5	NA
CG12453 (A8Y595)	0.93	3.0	1	1	0	0	NA
Ugt36Bc (Q8SZD9)	1.00	5.0	4	87	2	2	NA
Ephrin (Q8ST77)	0.92	2.9	1	1	2	3	membrane
Tetraspanin 3A (Q9NB16)	1.00	4.3	3	81	5	4	membrane
CG5273 (Q9NF32)	0.99	2.3	1	8	1	0	NA
CG14629 (Q9NF33)	0.99	3.1	1	3	1	0	NA
domeless (Q9VWE0)	1.00	5.1	7	51	2	1	membrane
CG30359 (Q8T0N3)	1.00	5.2	2	8	2	0	NA
lysosomal enzyme receptor protein (Q8IMR0)	1.00	1.2	3	13	1	2	membrane
LpR2 (Q7YTZ6)	0.98	1.9	1	2	1	1	membrane
CG31120 (Q86NX1)	0.99	1.9	1	50	2	2	NA
CG31195 (Q8IN49)	1.00	5.6	7	75	2	2	NA

Protein Name	PP	COV	num unique peps	tot num peps	Sosui TM	TM HMM	GO: cellular component
Neu3 (Q6QU65)	1.00	2.9	2	10	3	2	NA
CG32155 (Q8IQM9)	1.00	8.0	6	155	1	0	NA
CG32158 (Q8IQN6)	1.00	2.1	4	28	10	11	membrane
CG32594 (Q8MRG2)	1.00	4.1	4	66	2	1	NA
CG33087 (Q8MKP7)	1.00	6.9	38	378	2	1	membrane
CG33129 (Q9VKM7)	1.00	8.9	4	111	1	0	NA
CG33303 (Q8IH64)	1.00	8.3	11	236	2	2	membrane
Calcium activated protein for secretion (Q9NHE5)	1.00	8.0	4	19	0	0	membrane
CG40084 (Q7PLN5)	1.00	1.9	2	4	4	5	NA
(Q9VCG8)	0.99	1.4	1	16	1	1	NA
Organic cation transporter 2 (Q95R48)	1.00	8.5	17	118	10	12	membrane

Supplementary Table S4.2 List of glycoproteins monitored upon different stimuli. For each protein the ratio, the standard deviation (SD), the P-Value as well as the number of peptides quantified (num peps) for the different stimuli are listed.

Protein Name	LPS stimulated				Rapamycin stimulated				Vanadate stimulated			
	JRatio mean	JRatio SD	JRatio P-val	num peps	JRatio mean	JRatio SD	JRatio P-val	num peps	JRatio mean	JRatio SD	JRatio P-val	num peps
CG10221	0.61	0.26	0.02	1	0.54	0.19	<0.01	1	0.27	0.08	<0.01	1
Contactin (CG1084)	1.30	0.21	0.19	2	1.01	0.10	0.75	2	1.27	0.19	0.78	2
PTP 69D (CG10975)	1.84	0.47	<0.01	2	1.00	0.15	0.70	2	1.96	0.40	0.32	2
plexin A (CG11081)	0.86	0.06	0.51	1	0.47	0.16	<0.01	1	0.77	0.11	0.07	1
nicotinic acetylcholine receptor (CG11822)	0.88	0.07	0.58	1	0.96	0.06	0.50	1	0.93	0.06	0.22	1
Calnexin 99A (CG11958)	1.20	0.11	0.36	1	1.15	0.05	0.52	1	1.37	0.14	0.95	1
cueball (CG12086)	1.13	0.11	0.53	1	1.04	0.08	0.92	1	1.85	0.12	0.41	1
roundabout (CG13521)	1.97	0.29	<0.01	1	NA	NA	NA	NA	1.49	0.26	0.86	1
torso (CG1389)	1.02	0.04	0.89	1	0.93	0.04	0.39	1	0.82	0.03	0.12	2
CG14225	0.81	0.22	0.33	5	0.88	0.12	0.22	5	1.21	0.25	0.66	5
Eph RTK (CG1511)	1.36	0.17	0.13	1	0.97	0.15	0.55	1	1.76	0.22	0.49	1
Integrin b-PS (CG1560)	0.95	0.04	0.85	1	1.17	0.32	0.45	1	1.32	0.04	0.86	1
CG15744	1.46	0.31	0.06	2	1.11	0.21	0.70	2	1.92	0.40	0.35	2
CG16771	0.80	0.19	0.31	3	1.22	0.19	0.31	3	1.20	0.28	0.65	3
CG17667	1.13	0.13	0.51	2	1.16	0.12	0.49	2	1.43	0.20	0.95	2
Integrin (CG1771)	0.82	0.10	0.37	2	0.98	0.13	0.62	1	1.50	0.01	0.84	1
InR (CG18402)	1.05	0.07	0.78	3	0.97	0.06	0.57	6	1.48	0.10	0.87	4
CG2493	0.92	0.21	0.71	1	1.35	0.17	0.08	1	2.05	0.24	0.26	1
CG2791	0.89	0.09	0.62	2	1.17	0.08	0.47	1	1.69	0.08	0.57	1
halfway (CG3095)	1.21	0.13	0.33	1	1.17	0.09	0.46	1	2.04	0.18	0.27	1
Hydroxylase (CG31022)	1.08	0.14	0.66	3	1.17	0.14	0.45	3	1.40	0.15	0.99	3
CG31195	1.12	0.32	0.56	1	1.22	0.18	0.30	1	2.21	0.41	0.18	1
Basigin (CG31605)	0.86	0.03	0.51	8	1.10	0.03	0.77	8	1.17	0.04	0.59	9
CG31731	0.47	0.06	<0.01	1	1.03	0.15	0.86	3	0.75	0.10	0.06	2
CG31886	NA	NA	NA	NA	0.88	0.30	0.20	1	NA	NA	NA	NA
Transporter (CG31911)	0.65	0.06	0.04	2	0.86	0.06	0.16	2	1.65	0.17	0.63	2
CG32155	0.89	0.04	0.60	1	1.03	0.08	0.91	1	1.17	0.06	0.60	1
CG32594	NA	NA	NA	NA	0.52	0.00	<0.01	1	NA	NA	NA	NA
CG33087	1.16	0.16	0.44	4	1.19	0.12	0.40	4	1.70	0.12	0.57	4
CG33129	0.78	0.22	0.26	1	1.42	0.19	0.04	1	2.40	0.18	0.11	1
CG33303	0.67	0.13	0.06	1	0.79	0.16	0.05	1	1.17	0.17	0.60	2
unzipped (CG3533)	0.83	0.14	0.40	3	0.99	0.15	0.67	3	0.91	0.10	0.20	2
Fasciclin 2 (CG3665)	0.83	0.14	0.39	1	1.13	0.22	0.60	1	1.08	0.18	0.44	1
Tetraspanin (CG4591)	NA	NA	NA	NA	0.84	0.13	0.12	1	0.96	0.28	0.27	1
CG4726	NA	NA	NA	NA	NA	NA	NA	NA	0.94	0.10	0.24	1
CG4829	0.70	0.03	0.10	3	1.05	0.05	0.96	3	1.16	0.05	0.57	3
CG5284	1.04	0.21	0.81	1	0.65	0.14	<0.01	1	1.15	0.28	0.56	1
CG5594	1.16	0.09	0.44	1	1.10	1.06	0.77	2	1.92	0.05	0.35	2
CG5708	1.60	0.18	0.02	1	1.34	0.18	0.09	1	0.94	0.14	0.24	1
NPC-1 (CG5722)	0.53	0.04	<0.01	2	0.94	0.09	0.43	3	0.85	0.04	0.14	3
Tenascin (CG5723)	1.32	0.24	0.17	1	1.01	0.14	0.75	1	1.53	0.23	0.78	1
CG5789	0.96	0.24	0.89	1	1.35	0.14	0.08	1	2.60	0.40	0.07	1
Fasciclin 1 (CG6588)	0.90	0.18	0.65	4	1.26	0.25	0.21	4	1.13	0.17	0.52	3
Cad87A (CG6977)	1.34	0.41	0.15	1	1.74	0.40	<0.01	1	0.98	0.27	0.30	1

Supplemental Material

Protein Name	LPS stimulated				Rapamycin stimulated				Vanadate stimulated			
	JRatio mean	JRatio SD	JRatio P-val	num peps	JRatio mean	JRatio SD	JRatio P-val	num peps	JRatio mean	JRatio SD	JRatio P-val	num peps
Laminin B1 (CG7123)	0.81	0.09	0.34	1	1.42	0.45	0.04	1	1.13	0.16	0.52	1
kuzbanian (CG7147)	1.11	0.09	0.57	1	1.23	0.17	0.28	2	1.40	0.13	1.00	1
peste (CG7228)	1.10	0.23	0.63	1	0.94	0.16	0.43	1	1.13	0.22	0.53	1
Macroglobulin (CG7586)	0.99	0.09	1.00	1	1.36	0.14	0.07	1	1.13	0.14	0.52	1
CG7800	0.99	0.20	0.99	4	1.02	0.10	0.83	4	1.86	0.29	0.40	4
Integrin (CG8095)	1.20	0.24	0.36	1	1.28	0.20	0.17	1	1.37	0.23	0.95	1
PDGF/VEGF (CG8222)	0.99	0.02	0.99	1	0.90	0.04	0.27	1	1.42	0.03	0.97	1
CG8486	1.46	0.56	0.06	1	0.92	0.31	0.34	1	1.43	0.47	0.95	1
frazzled (CG8581)	NA	NA	NA	NA	1.44	0.31	0.03	1	1.70	0.41	0.56	1
Cirl (CG8639)	1.10	0.15	0.60	1	1.07	0.10	0.92	1	1.18	0.13	0.62	1
G-cyclase (CG8742)	0.36	0.17	<0.01	2	0.60	0.17	<0.01	2	0.45	0.14	<0.01	2
Proteinase (CG8947)	1.90	0.52	<0.01	1	2.09	0.46	<0.01	1	2.88	0.42	0.03	1
nervana 1 (CG9258)	1.19	0.16	0.38	1	0.91	0.05	0.30	1	0.77	0.13	0.08	1
Neurotactin (CG9704)	0.91	0.23	0.70	1	1.00	0.12	0.70	1	0.97	0.16	0.28	1
CG9917	1.14	0.27	0.49	1	1.06	0.13	0.95	1	1.56	0.12	0.75	1
CG9947	0.92	0.18	0.72	1	0.99	0.14	0.66	1	0.86	0.14	0.15	1
CG9953	NA	NA	NA	NA	NA	NA	NA	NA	0.79	0.10	0.09	1

Supplementary Table S4.3 List of glycoproteins identified quantified in the insulin stimulation experiment using CSC. For each protein the ratio, the standard deviation (SD), the P-Value as well as the number of peptides quantified JRatio are listed. Protein entries shown in bold were detected in both the CSC and whole membrane capturing experiment and are depicted in Figure 4.7d.

Protein Name	JRatio mean	JRatio SD	JRatio P-value	peptides quantified
Saposin-related	0.81	0.38	0.96	1
Fasciclin 1	0.87	0.34	0.91	7
halfway	1.00	0.19	0.67	8
Laminin B1	1.26	0.31	0.33	1
Integrin alpha-PS3	1.20	0.58	0.38	1
Protein tyrosine phosphatase 4E	1.10	0.40	0.52	1
Tenascin major	0.99	0.44	0.69	2
Integrin alpha-PS1	1.03	0.66	0.63	1
Integrin beta-PS	0.91	0.37	0.83	4
roundabout	2.73	0.68	<0.01	1
cueball	0.61	0.24	0.48	6
Basigin	0.86	0.36	0.94	10
frazzled	0.29	0.34	<0.01	2
Insulin receptor	0.41	0.07	0.09	6
Protein tyrosine phosphatase 69D	0.62	0.20	0.50	3
Calnexin 99A	0.77	0.25	0.87	2
kuzbanian	0.63	0.12	0.52	7
Niemann-Pick Type C-1	0.60	0.09	0.45	9
plexin A	0.82	0.14	0.98	3
Equilibrative nucleoside transporter 2	1.01	0.20	0.65	1
lethal (1) G0289	0.61	0.15	0.46	1
26-29kD-proteinase	0.83	0.28	1.00	1
CG15347	0.84	0.24	1.00	2
CG9947	0.64	0.37	0.55	2
CG4829	1.00	0.20	0.69	3
CG14225	1.36	0.19	0.25	6
CG1518	0.33	0.09	0.01	2
nicotinic acetylcholine receptor beta 21C	1.11	0.45	0.50	1
CG8486	1.00	0.38	0.69	4
PDGF- and VEGF-receptor related	0.97	0.49	0.73	5
CG4972	0.60	0.11	0.43	1
CG16771	0.48	0.15	0.20	2
CG2493	1.02	0.26	0.63	1
CG3305	0.87	0.28	0.91	1
gp210	0.95	0.18	0.77	1
Tetraspanin 42EI	0.21	0.15	<0.01	1
Cirl	1.38	0.37	0.23	3

Supplemental Material

Protein Name	JRatio mean	JRatio SD	JRatio P-value	peptides quantified
lambik	1.38	0.23	0.23	2
CG3907	1.06	0.42	0.59	1
wntless	1.34	0.41	0.25	1
CG17667	1.09	0.28	0.53	3
fat2	0.87	0.17	0.91	2
CG3618	1.33	0.07	0.26	1
Contactin	0.79	0.27	0.91	4
CG2791	0.95	0.37	0.77	2
CG7800	0.96	0.34	0.75	6
CG8507	0.93	0.37	0.79	1
Cad87A	1.15	0.56	0.45	1
CG9796	0.91	0.12	0.85	1
CG5789	1.21	0.27	0.38	1
CG32158	0.38	0.17	0.05	2
CG33087	1.27	0.16	0.33	15
CG33129	0.51	0.15	0.24	2
CG33303	1.25	0.27	0.34	3
CG40084	0.85	0.32	0.96	2
Neuroglian	0.51	0.29	0.25	1
punt	0.65	0.47	0.57	1
unzipped	1.05	0.22	0.59	4
Neurotactin	0.67	0.38	0.61	1
lethal (2) 08717	1.06	0.30	0.57	1
Sema-1a	1.45	0.33	0.19	1
Sema-2a	1.32	0.22	0.27	1
Oligosaccharyl transferase 3	0.36	0.05	0.03	1
division abnormally delayed	1.05	0.23	0.59	1
Gp150	0.37	0.22	0.05	1
nervana 2	0.92	0.37	0.81	1
Macroglobulin complement-related	0.51	0.22	0.25	3
CG5594	1.34	0.32	0.26	4
plexin B	1.02	0.43	0.65	2
Eph receptor tyrosine kinase	1.09	0.85	0.53	1
prominin-like	0.70	0.27	0.69	2
CG3638	0.48	0.11	0.20	1
CG31731	1.13	0.34	0.46	2
dispatched	2.44	0.14	<0.01	1
Tollo	1.01	0.23	0.65	1
Hemolectin	0.99	0.16	0.69	4
CG17660	0.64	0.41	0.53	1
CG9027	1.15	0.37	0.45	1
straightjacket	1.69	0.18	0.08	1
Dystroglycan	0.45	0.17	0.14	1
CG11961	0.47	0.14	0.17	2
Organic anion transporting polypeptide 58Dc	0.53	0.13	0.29	3
CG7638	0.89	0.19	0.89	2
CG5284	1.10	0.27	0.52	1
Adenosine deaminase-related growth factor A	1.52	0.15	0.15	2
CG5976	1.09	0.21	0.53	1
Tetraspanin 86D	0.88	0.24	0.91	2
CG14857	2.00	0.41	0.02	1
CG17119	2.08	0.52	0.01	1
nicastrin	0.47	0.19	0.18	1
CG14516	1.24	0.73	0.35	1
Ugt36Bc	0.51	0.19	0.25	2
Tetraspanin 3A	1.05	0.39	0.59	1
domeless	0.88	0.25	0.89	2
CG30359	1.37	0.39	0.24	1
CG31120	0.51	0.36	0.25	1
CG31195	0.99	0.23	0.69	1
CG32155	0.90	0.50	0.85	2
CG32594	1.06	0.44	0.57	1
Calcium activated protein for secretion	0.99	0.21	0.69	2
Organic cation transporter 2	2.52	0.18	<0.01	1

Supplemental Material

Supplementary Table S4.4 ICPL labeling results of glycoproteins identified quantified in the insulin stimulation experiment. Protein ratios and standard deviation (SD) obtained by XPRESS from isotopically labeled peptides are shown including protein probability (PP) and protein coverage (COV).

Protein Name	PP	COV	XPRESS mean	XPRESS SD	XPRESS num peptides	num unique peptides	tot num peptides
CG3305	1.00	3.1	1.06	0.07	4	1	4
CG2213	1.00	2.8	1.27	0.05	3	1	7
CG9796	1.00	5.2	0.82	0.03	2	1	4
Ribosomal protein L18	1.00	4.3	0.92	0.10	2	2	3
CG9917	1.00	3.0	1.48	0.08	2	1	2
CG2791	1.00	2.8	0.99	0.12	8	4	16
domeless	1.00	1.2	0.88	0.09	2	1	4
Protein tyrosine phosphatase 69D	1.00	1.2	0.63	0.01	2	2	5
cueball	1.00	4.3	0.85	0.01	2	2	7
Protein tyrosine phosphatase 4E	1.00	0.7	0.89	0.01	2	1	4
yolkless	1.00	1.1	0.81	0.00	1	2	3
CG5594	1.00	0.8	0.65	0.03	4	1	8
Integrin beta-PS	1.00	0.9	0.85	0.00	3	1	6
nicotinic acetylcholine receptor beta 21C	1.00	3.1	1.02	0.04	4	1	7
Insulin receptor	1.00	2.1	0.42	0.08	9	5	16
CG33309	1.00	3.4	15.74	0.98	2	3	3
CG4726	1.00	3.5	0.50	0.11	4	1	4
CG10353	1.00	0.9	0.94	0.07	2	1	4
Basigin	1.00	19.6	1.07	0.13	22	13	49
Organic cation transporter 2	1.00	2.7	0.86	0.08	3	2	7
Tenascin major	1.00	0.7	1.13	0.05	2	2	5
Sug	1.00	1.7	0.98	0.01	2	2	4
frazzled	1.00	1.7	1.51	0.14	3	1	4
CG8029	1.00	2.1	1.13	0.05	4	1	8
CG10795	1.00	3.9	0.99	0.00	2	1	3
plexin A	1.00	1.9	-9.90	-9.90	0	1	2
CG32155	1.00	5.6	1.17	0.03	2	2	6
CG7800	1.00	4.7	-9.90	-9.90	0	2	3
CG5976	1.00	3.1	0.57	0.02	2	1	4
CG33087	1.00	0.8	1.01	0.04	3	3	6
Integrin alpha-PS3	1.00	1.7	0.91	0.27	3	1	4
Niemann-Pick Type C-1	1.00	1.5	0.86	0.05	5	2	11
Integrin alpha-PS1	1.00	0.8	1.53	0.22	4	1	4
nervana 1	1.00	4.9	0.99	0.09	3	3	9
Macroglobulin complement-related	1.00	1.1	0.93	0.10	4	3	7
Activin receptor	1.00	2.1	0.89	0.03	2	1	4
Equilibrative nucleoside transporter 2	0.99	3.1	1.94	0.00	1	1	3
CG32594	0.99	1.5	1.19	0.17	2	1	4
CG3638	0.99	1.3	0.55	0.04	2	1	4
CG14516	0.99	1.5	1.16	0.04	2	1	4
CG14225	0.98	1.1	0.87	0.17	3	1	3
Contactin	0.93	0.9	-9.90	-9.90	0	1	1

Supplementary Table S4.5 List of glycoproteins identified quantified in the insulin stimulation experiment using whole membrane glycocapturing. For each protein the ratio, the standard deviation (SD), the *P*-value as well as the number of peptides quantified by JRatio are listed. Protein entries shown in bold were detected in both the CSC and whole membrane capturing experiment and are depicted in Figure 4.7d.

Protein Name	JRatio mean	JRatio SD	JRatio *P*-value	n peptides quantified
Saposin-related	1.24	0.22	0.05	3
Fasciclin 1	0.99	0.48	0.23	2
halfway	1.66	0.37	0.05	1
Laminin B1	1.35	0.33	0.05	3
Integrin alpha-PS3	0.82	0.19	0.91	1
Protein tyrosine phosphatase 4E	0.46	0.24	0.05	1
Tenascin major	0.98	0.20	0.30	1
Integrin alpha-PS1	1.03	0.37	0.17	1
Integrin beta-PS	0.99	0.25	0.23	3
roundabout	1.43	0.89	0.05	1
cueball	1.30	0.62	0.05	1
Basigin	0.83	0.14	0.82	5
frazzled	0.87	0.32	0.63	1
Insulin receptor	0.94	0.24	0.38	2
Protein tyrosine phosphatase 69D	0.54	0.08	0.05	2
Calnexin 99A	0.99	0.63	0.23	1
kuzbanian	0.93	0.40	0.38	1
Niemann-Pick Type C-1	0.45	0.05	0.05	2
plexin A	0.87	0.15	0.63	6
Equilibrative nucleoside transporter 2	0.74	0.14	0.72	1
lethal (1) G0289	1.76	0.33	0.05	4
26-29kD-proteinase	1.11	0.19	0.05	1
CG15347	0.72	0.07	0.63	1
CG9947	0.62	0.08	0.11	1
CG4829	1.00	0.34	0.23	2
CG14225	0.67	0.15	0.30	7
CG1518	0.87	0.11	0.63	1
nicotinic acetylcholine receptor beta 21C	0.88	0.13	0.63	1
CG8486	0.77	0.23	0.82	1
PDGF- and VEGF-receptor related	1.00	0.25	0.23	1
CG4972	0.97	0.25	0.30	2
CG16771	0.48	0.17	0.05	1
CG2493	0.85	0.12	0.72	4
CG3305	0.99	0.24	0.23	2
gp210	0.48	0.07	0.05	1
Tetraspanin 42EI	1.01	0.34	0.12	2
Cirl	1.23	0.42	0.05	2
lambik	1.69	0.74	0.05	1
CG3907	0.92	0.42	0.46	1
wntless	0.55	0.04	0.05	1
CG17667	0.91	0.21	0.55	1
fat2	0.72	0.27	0.55	1
CG3618	1.05	0.36	0.11	1
Contactin	0.83	0.26	0.82	1
CG2791	0.82	0.26	0.91	2
CG7800	0.81	0.16	0.91	5
CG8507	0.93	0.31	0.38	1
Cad87A	0.64	0.13	0.23	2
CG9796	0.76	0.07	0.72	1
CG5789	0.68	0.25	0.38	2
CG32158	0.92	0.44	0.43	1
CG33087	0.93	0.13	0.46	6
CG33129	0.91	0.27	0.46	1
CG33303	0.95	0.58	0.38	1
CG40084	0.87	0.19	0.63	1
Fasciclin 2	0.59	0.12	0.05	2
inflated	1.07	0.22	0.05	1
Laminin A	1.09	0.27	0.05	3
off-track	0.44	0.11	0.05	1
Guanylyl cyclase at 76C	0.68	0.16	0.38	2
kekkon-1	0.98	0.57	0.23	2
Tyrosine-protein kinase receptor torso	1.86	0.11	0.05	1

Supplemental Material

Protein Name	JRatio mean	JRatio SD	JRatio P-value	n peptides quantified
CG2918	0.84	0.20	0.82	1
CG3975	0.25	0.14	0.05	1
CG10221	0.94	0.46	0.38	1
CG7453	1.21	0.43	0.05	1
interference Hedgehog	0.62	0.14	0.11	1
peste	0.98	0.69	0.23	1
CadN2	0.86	0.29	0.72	1
CG10702	0.74	0.15	0.63	1
CG16868	0.65	0.21	0.23	1
CG7739	1.35	0.23	0.05	1
CG5235	0.98	0.29	0.30	1
CG3303	0.49	0.13	0.05	1
CG7702	0.45	0.07	0.05	1
CG6490	0.84	0.22	0.82	1
prolyl-4-hydroxylase-alpha EFB	0.94	0.53	0.38	1
CG34355	0.80	0.37	0.91	1

Supplementary Table S5.1 List of glycoproteins selected as potential *Pten* dependant prostate cancer markers identified by in-depth MS based proteomic analysis. Protein ratios measured by either elution profile comparison or spectral counting of $Pten^{-/-}$ (n=3) and $Pten^{+/+}$ (n=3) mouse tissue at 8 and 18 weeks of age. The regulations are indicated by either up in cancer (up), down in cancer (down), or detected only in cancer bearing mice (Ca only) including the *P*-Value.

			8 weeks old mice				18 weeks old mice			
			Elution profile		Spectral counting		Elution profile		Spectral counting	
UniProt ID	Protein Name	Ratio-nale*	cancer/control	P-Val	cancer/control	P-Val	cancer/control	P-Val	cancer/control	P-Val
Q9D7N9	Adipocyte PM-associated protein	1	up	0.02	up	0.19	up	0.85	down	0.50
P28653	Biglycan	1	down	0.69	up	0.28	up	0.99	up	0.08
Q00493	Carboxypeptidase E	1	up	0.12	up	0.19	-	-	-	-
Q80V42	Carboxypeptidase M	1	-	-	up	0.10	up	0.49	up	0.03
P31809	CEA-rel. cell adhesion molecule 1	1, 4	up	0.56	up	0.01	up	0.97	up	0.08
P70269	Cathepsin E	1, 4	-	-	up	0.13	-	-	up	0.21
Q8R5M8	Cell adhesion molecule 1	1	up	0.01	down	0.45	up	0.19	up	0.32
Q06890	Clusterin	1, 4	up	0.26	up	<0.01	up	0.04	up	-
P11087	Collagen alpha-1(I) chain	1	-	-	-	-	-	-	up	0.01
Q63870	Collagen alpha-1(VII) chain	1	-	-	-	-	up	0.52	up	0.05
Q80X19	Collagen alpha-1(XIV) chain	1	-	-	up	0.42	-	-	up	0.10
P04186	Complement factor B	1, 4	-	-	down	0.19	up	0.21	up	0.03
P06909	Complement factor H	1, 4	up	0.63	down	0.35	up	0.03	up	0.02
O35649	Cyclophilin C-associated protein	1, 4	up	0.21	up	0.01	up	0.02	up	<0.01
Q62287	Cyritestin	1, 4	up	0.26	up	0.12	-	-	up	0.07
Q60997	Deleted in brain tumors 1 protein	1	-	-	-	-	up	0.93	up	0.04
Q8R242	Di-N-acetylchitobiase	1	-	-	-	-	Ca only	<0.01	up	0.01
Q9ET22	Dipeptidyl-peptidase 2	1, 4	-	-	-	-	up	0.13	up	0.01
Q99K41	EMILIN-1	1	up	0.13	up	0.29	up	0.75	down	0.36
Q9EQH2	ER aminopeptidase 1	1	-	-	up	0.19	up	0.69	up	0.04
Q3UVK0	ER metallopeptidase 1	1	up	<0.01	up	0.05	up	0.01	up	<0.01
Q01279	Epidermal growth factor receptor	1, 4	up	0.23	down	0.19	up	0.06	up	0.05
Q61508	Extracellular matrix protein 1	1	-	-	-	-	up	0.07	up	0.04
Q61554	Fibrillin-1	1	up	0.21	up	0.11	up	0.09	up	0.01
P11276	Fibronectin	1, 4	up	0.11	up	0.07	up	0.80	up	0.14
Q8VEB1	G protein-coupled receptor kinase 5	1, 7	down	0.66	up	0.05	-	-	-	-
Q9Z0L8	Gamma-glutamyl hydrolase	1, 4	-	-	-	-	Ca only	<0.01	up	0.02
Q91XA2	Golgi phosphoprotein 2	1	up	0.42	up	0.19	up	0.01	up	0.09
Q6PD26	GPI transamidase component PIG-S	1	up	0.28	up	0.03	up	0.52	up	0.29
P01869	IGG-1 chain C membrane-bound.	1, 4	down	0.69	up	0.39	up	0.04	up	0.07
P43406	Integrin alpha-V	1, 4	up	0.69	up	0.35	up	0.60	up	0.02
Q91XL1	Leucine-rich alpha-2-glycoprotein	1, 4	-	-	down	0.19	Ca only	<0.01	up	0.01
P51885	Lumican	1, 4	up	0.31	up	0.42	up	0.87	up	0.03
O09159	Lysosomal alpha-mannosidase	1, 4	-	-	up	0.19	up	0.84	up	0.15
P16675	Lysosomal protective protein	1, 4	up	0.60	up	0.04	up	0.83	down	0.32
P11438	Lamp-1	1	-	-	up	0.02	up	0.98	up	0.20

Supplemental Material

UniProt ID	Protein Name	Rationale*	8 weeks old mice				18 weeks old mice			
			Elution profile		Spectral counting		Elution profile		Spectral counting	
			cancer/ control	P-Val	cancer/ control	P-Val	cancer/ control	P-Val	cancer/ control	P-Val
P17047	Lamp-2	1	up	0.66	up	0.08	up	0.59	up	0.20
P12032	Metalloproteinase inhibitor 1	1	-	-	-	-	up	0.31	up	0.01
Q9D1H9	Microfibril-associated glycoprotein 4	1, 4	down	0.63	up	0.33	up	0.94	up	0.08
Q61903	Myeloid secondary granule protein	1	Ca only	<0.01	up	0.05	Ca only	<0.01	up	0.03
Q3UZZ4	Olfactomedin-4	1	-	-	up	0.19	-	-	up	0.12
Q3UQ28	Peroxidasin homolog	1	up	<0.01	up	0.19	up	0.44	up	0.14
Q9WVJ3	Plasma glutamate carboxypeptidase	1, 4	up	<0.01	up	0.04	up	0.21	up	0.02
P97290	Plasma protease C1 inhibitor	1, 4	Ca only	<0.01	down	0.19	Ca only	<0.01	up	<0.01
O70570	Polymeric-immunoglobulin receptor	1	up	<0.01	up	0.02	up	<0.01	up	0.01
P15501	Prostatic spermine-binding protein	1, 7	up	0.15	down	0.21	-	-	-	-
P97805	Protein FAM3D	1	down	0.63	up	0.21	up	0.03	up	0.12
Q8VCI0	Putative phospholipase B-like 1	1, 4	-	-	-	-	Ca only	<0.01	up	0.01
Q64455	Receptor-type tyr-phosphatase eta	1	-	-	-	-	up	0.94	up	0.05
Q8CEK3	Ser protease inhibitor protein	1	up	0.79	up	0.14	-	-	up	0.21
Q60854	Serpin B6	1	up	0.14	down	0.19	-	-	-	-
Q62087	Serum paraoxonase/lactonase 3	1	up	0.11	up	0.19	up	0.05	up	0.02
Q5K5D4	Spink5 protein	1	-	-	-	-	up	0.62	up	0.03
Q8BND5	Sulfhydryl oxidase 1	1, 4	-	-	-	-	Ca only	<0.01	up	0.01
Q80YX1	Tenascin	1	-	-	-	-	-	-	up	0.10
Q99J59	Tetraspanin 1	1, 7	up	0.01	up	0.09	up	0.16	up	0.05
P35441	Thrombospondin-1	1, 4	Ca only	<0.01	up	0.02	Ca only	<0.01	up	<0.01
P01831	Thy-1 membrane glycoprotein	1	up	0.02	up	0.17	up	0.31	up	0.08
Q8R3G9	Tspan8	1	up	0.53	up	0.13	up	0.05	up	0.01
O88493	Type VI collagen alpha 3 subunit	1	up	0.07	up	0.28	up	0.90	down	0.44
Q62059	Versican core protein	1	-	-	up	0.35	up	0.44	up	0.09
P20029	78 kDa glucose-regulated protein	2, 4	-	-	-	-	-	-	down	0.10
Q8VHH7	Adenylate cyclase type 3	2, 4	-	-	-	-	-	-	down	0.01
P97449	Aminopeptidase N	2, 4	up	0.26	down	0.10	up	0.62	up	0.27
Q6TU36	Beta-defensin 50	2	down	0.11	up	0.45	down	<0.01	down	0.05
O08540	Beta-microseminoprotein	2, 7	down	0.01	down	0.13	down	<0.01	down	0.04
Q61400	CEACAM 10	2	down	0.60	down	0.43	down	0.02	down	0.27
P18242	Cathepsin D	2, 4	down	0.53	down	0.45	up	0.55	down	0.10
Q9CYA0	Cys-rich with EGF-domain protein	2, 7	-	-	down	0.10	down	<0.01	down	0.03
P28843	Dipeptidyl peptidase 4	2	down	0.90	up	0.40	up	0.75	down	0.15
P08113	Endoplasmin	2, 4	down	0.18	down	0.24	down	0.01	down	0.02
P17439	Glucosylceramidase	2	down	0.93	down	0.23	up	0.82	down	0.15
Q8CDQ9	Hypothetical Glycoside hydrolase	2	-	-	down	0.04	-	-	-	-
Q8BZG2	von Willebrand factor type D protein	2, 4	up	0.42	down	0.36	down	<0.01	down	0.01
Q9JKR6	Hypoxia up-regulated protein 1	2	down	0.15	down	0.15	down	0.01	down	<0.01
Q8BJD1	Inter-alpha-trypsin inhibitor	2	-	-	up	0.50	down	0.30	down	0.01
P19137	Laminin subunit alpha-1	2	-	-	down	0.19	down	0.35	down	0.03
Q60675	Laminin subunit alpha-2	2	down	0.20	down	0.09	down	0.38	up	0.30
P97927	Laminin subunit alpha-4	2	down	0.35	down	0.13	down	0.22	down	0.10
P02469	Laminin subunit beta-1	2	-	-	down	0.10	down	0.41	down	0.23
P02468	Laminin subunit gamma-1	2	down	0.96	down	0.43	down	0.41	down	0.14
A1L0S2	LOC100037259 protein	2	-	-	-	-	down	<0.01	down	0.03
Q91ZX7	LLR-related protein 1	2, 4	down	0.13	up	0.30	up	0.66	up	-
O70423	Membrane copper amine oxidase	2	down	0.60	down	0.19	down	0.02	down	0.04
P11627	Neural cell adhesion molecule L1	2, 4	-	-	down	0.09	-	-	down	0.25
P97300	Neuroplastin	2, 4	-	-	up	0.19	up	0.15	down	0.36
Q5BKQ4	Pancreatic lipase-related protein 1	2	down	0.28	down	0.17	down	<0.01	down	0.08
P70208	Plexin 3	2	up	0.63	down	0.10	down	0.01	down	0.11
O54990	Prominin-1	2, 4	down	0.79	down	0.28	up	0.98	down	0.11
O88668	Protein CREG1	2	up	0.79	down	0.28	down	0.14	down	0.25
Q3UN54	Secreted seminal-vesicle protein	2, 4	down	0.90	up	0.27	down	0.10	down	0.25
Q64367	Seminal vesicle autoantigen	2	down	0.79	up	0.22	down	0.05	up	0.32
Q92II1	Serotransferrin	2, 4	-	-	down	0.13	up	0.59	up	0.21
Q14AE4	Wap four-disulfide core domain 3	2	-	-	down	0.06	up	<0.01	down	0.01
Q8BM27	Weakly similar to LYSOZYME C	2	down	0.40	up	0.43	down	0.06	down	0.01
Q8CIF4	Biotinidase	3, 4	down	0.86	down	0.14	up	0.13	down	0.16
Q60847	Collagen alpha-1(XII) chain	3, 4	down	0.86	down	0.13	up	0.10	-	-
Q8BZE1	hypothetical Speract receptor	3, 7	up	0.28	up	0.08	down	0.06	down	0.27
P42703	Leukemia inhibitory factor receptor	3, 4	up	0.20	down	0.13	up	0.01	up	0.35
Q9JK53	Prolargin	3	up	0.69	down	0.12	up	0.16	up	0.02
P00683	Ribonuclease pancreatic	3	down	0.83	up	0.08	down	0.02	down	0.06
P09036	Serine protease inhibitor Kazal-type	3, 7	-	-	up	0.11	-	-	down	0.07

Supplemental Material

UniProt ID	Protein Name	Rationale*	8 weeks old mice				18 weeks old mice			
			Elution profile		Spectral counting		Elution profile		Spectral counting	
			cancer/control	P-Val	cancer/control	P-Val	cancer/control	P-Val	cancer/control	P-Val
P14231	Na/K-transporting ATPase	3, 4	down	0.45	up	0.07	down	0.21	down	0.01
P22967	Angiotensin-converting enzyme	4	up	0.66	down	0.36	up	0.63	down	0.26
P15379	CD44 antigen	4	-	-	up	0.19	-	-	-	-
Q61147	Ceruloplasmin	4	-	-	down	0.18	-	-	-	-
Q9CQE7	ER-Golgi inter compartment protein	4	-	-	up	0.47	up	0.57	down	0.18
P35922	Fragile X mental retardation protein	4	-	-	-	-	-	-	up	0.21
Q9QYE6	Golgin subfamily A member 5	4	down	0.93	up	0.19	-	-	-	-
P28798	Granulins	4	-	-	-	-	-	-	up	0.21
P01897	H-2 class I histocompatibility antigen	4	-	-	up	0.19	-	-	-	-
Q61646	Haptoglobin	4	-	-	down	0.19	-	-	up	0.21
P09055	Integrin beta-1	4	down	0.90	up	0.47	up	0.75	down	0.28
Q61789	Laminin subunit alpha-3	4	-	-	-	-	up	0.69	down	0.38
P04939	Major urinary protein 3	4	-	-	-	-	-	-	-	-
Q61391	Neprilysin	4	down	0.86	up	0.44	up	0.78	down	0.37
P13594	Neural cell adhesion molecule 1	4	-	-	up	0.19	-	-	up	0.27
Q8CH77	Neuron navigator 1	4	down	0.66	up	0.19	-	-	-	-
Q14AV9	Pdia2 protein	4	-	-	-	-	-	-	-	-
Q62009	Periostin	4	-	-	-	-	-	-	up	0.21
P27773	Protein disulfide-isomerase A3	4	-	-	-	-	-	-	down	0.21
Q922R8	Protein disulfide-isomerase A6	4	-	-	-	-	-	-	down	0.21
O35204	Putative pheromone receptor	4	-	-	down	0.19	-	-	-	-
Q9WUP1	Receptor activity-modifying protien 3	4	-	-	up	0.19	-	-	-	-
Q9QVY8	Retinoic acid-induced protein 2	4	-	-	-	-	-	-	-	-
Q61207	Sulfated glycoprotein 1	4	-	-	up	0.39	-	-	up	0.21
Q62351	Transferrin receptor protein 1	4	-	-	-	-	-	-	up	0.21
P21614	Vitamin D-binding protein	4	-	-	-	-	-	-	-	-
P29788	Vitronectin	4	-	-	-	-	-	-	-	-
Q64726	Zinc-alpha-2-glycoprotein	4, 7	-	-	up	0.39	-	-	down	0.21
O08860	Agrin	5	up	0.76	up	0.25	up	0.72	down	0.46
Q99MQ4	Asporin	5	down	0.83	down	0.16	up	0.84	down	0.42
Q6XBG1	ATP-binding cassette transporter	5	-	-	-	-	-	-	down	0.21
Q0P6B3	BC023744 protein	5	-	-	-	-	-	-	-	-
A6H586	Collagen type VI alpha 5	5	-	-	-	-	down	0.23	down	0.25
Q9EQG7	Ectonucleotide pyrophosphatase	5	-	-	up	0.19	-	-	up	0.45
Q61001	Laminin subunit alpha-5	5	down	0.28	up	0.39	down	0.37	down	0.25
Q61292	Laminin subunit beta-2	5	-	-	up	0.19	-	-	-	-
Q3T998	A kinase (PRKA) anchor protein 13	6	-	-	-	-	-	-	-	-
Q9WV54	Acid ceramidase	6	-	-	-	-	-	-	up	0.18
Q8VBT6	Apolipoprotein B-100 receptor	6	-	-	-	-	-	-	-	-
Q6P8S1	Aspartate-beta-hydroxylase	6	-	-	-	-	down	0.41	up	0.44
Q9WU60	Attractin	6	-	-	-	-	-	-	up	0.32
O88783	Coagulation factor V	6	-	-	-	-	-	-	-	-
O08543	Ephrin-a5	6	-	-	up	0.19	up	0.71	down	0.46
Q8K2E1	G1 to S phase transition 1	6	-	-	-	-	-	-	-	-
Q60677	Integrin alpha-E	6	-	-	-	-	-	-	-	-
P05532	Mast/stem cell growth factor receptor	6	-	-	-	-	-	-	up	0.21
Q9JLI3	Membrane metallo-endopeptidase	6	-	-	up	0.17	up	0.92	up	0.28
P70232	Neural cell adhesion molecule L1	6	up	0.53	up	0.17	up	0.92	up	0.28
Q3UH76	Plexin B2	6	-	-	-	-	up	0.59	up	0.30
P01132	Pro-epidermal growth factor	6, 7	down	0.35	up	0.40	up	0.70	down	0.47
O08976	Probasin	6, 7	-	-	-	-	-	-	down	0.21
P28301	Protein-lysine 6-oxidase	6	-	-	-	-	-	-	-	-
Q8K1B9	N-acetylgalactosaminyltransferase	6	-	-	-	-	-	-	up	0.50
P35822	Receptor-type tyr-protein phosphatase.	6	-	-	up	0.19	-	-	-	-
O09126	Semaphorin-4D	6	-	-	-	-	-	-	-	-
P97321	Seprase	6	-	-	-	-	-	-	-	-
Q9ET90	Transmembrane 9 superfamily member 3	6	up	0.76	down	0.18	up	0.66	down	0.25
P29754	Type-1A angiotensin II receptor	6	-	-	-	-	-	-	-	-
P97797	Tyr-protein phosphatase substrate 1	6	-	-	-	-	-	-	up	0.20
P35917	VEGF receptor 3	6	-	-	-	-	-	-	-	-
Q9CZT5	Vasorin	6	-	-	-	-	-	-	-	-
O08532	Voltage-dependent calcium channel	6	-	-	-	-	-	-	down	0.21

* Rationales for choosing the different proteins. 1: up in cancer (61 proteins), 2: down in cancer (34), 3: regulated in cancer (8), 4: detected in serum, (69), 5: secreted protein (8), 6: prior knowledge (26) 7: prostate specific (10)

Supplemental Material

Supplementary Table S5.2 List of proteins analyzed by SRM in sera of $Pten^{-/-}$ (n=3) and $Pten^{+/+}$ (n=3) mice at 8 and 18 weeks of age. Displayed columns include the gene and protein name; the mean value of the protein concentration measured including the standard deviation (SD); the protein ratio and the P-Value.

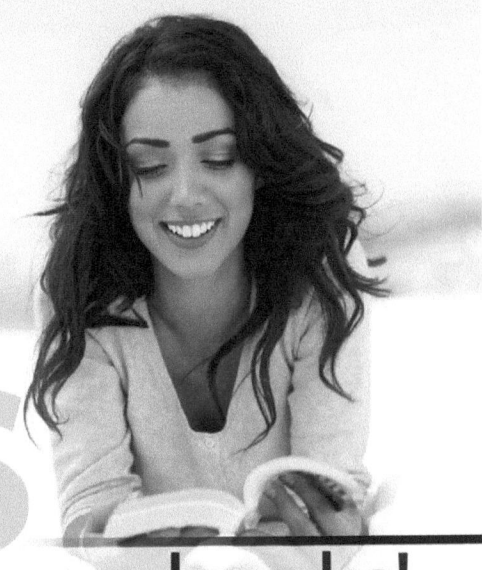

I want morebooks!

Buy your books fast and straightforward online - at one of the world's fastest growing online book stores! Environmentally sound due to Print-on-Demand technologies.

Buy your books online at
www.get-morebooks.com

Kaufen Sie Ihre Bücher schnell und unkompliziert online – auf einer der am schnellsten wachsenden Buchhandelsplattformen weltweit!
Dank Print-On-Demand umwelt- und ressourcenschonend produziert.

Bücher schneller online kaufen
www.morebooks.de

OmniScriptum Marketing DEU GmbH
Heinrich-Böcking-Str. 6-8
D - 66121 Saarbrücken
Telefax: +49 681 93 81 567-9

info@omniscriptum.com
www.omniscriptum.com

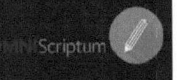

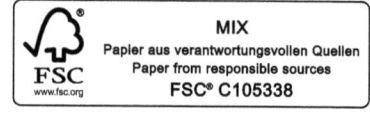

Printed by Books on Demand GmbH, Norderstedt / Germany